UROLOGY
Case Studies
Second Edition

A Compilation of 60 Clinical Studies

By   **BERNARD FRUCHTMAN, M.D.**
Associate Clinical Professor of Urology
Albert Einstein College of Medicine
Bronx, New York;
Attending Urologist
Beth Israel Medical Center
New York, New York;
Bronx Municipal Hospital Center
Bronx, New York

and

HARRY R. NEWMAN, M.D.
Professor and Chairman
Department of Urology
Albert Einstein College of Medicine
Bronx, New York

THE BRITISH SCHOOL OF OSTEOPATHY
1-4 SUFFOLK STREET, LONDON SW1Y 4HG
TEL: 01-930 9254-8

Copyright © 1979 by
MEDICAL EXAMINATION
PUBLISHING CO., INC.
an Excerpta Medica company

Library of Congress Card Number
79-88722

ISBN 0-87488-017-3

August, 1979

All rights reserved. No part of this
publication may be reproduced in any
form or by any means, electronic or
mechanical, including photocopy,
without permission in writing from
the publisher.

Printed in the United States of America

SIMULTANEOUSLY PUBLISHED IN:

Brazil	:	GUANABARA KOOGAN Rio de Janeiro, Brazil
Europe	:	HANS HUBER PUBLISHERS Bern, Switzerland
Japan	:	IGAKU-SHOIN Ltd. Tokyo, Japan
South and East Asia	:	TOPPAN COMPANY (S) Pte. Ltd. Singapore
United Kingdom	:	HENRY KIMPTON PUBLISHERS London, England

preface

The following urologic case histories are presented as a brief review of basic principles in urology, for the practitioner, resident, intern, and for those preparing for medical board examinations. The cases have been selected to demonstrate basic principles of management. The text as a whole emphasizes day-to-day patient care; it is intended to serve as a practically oriented clinical review rather than an exhaustive discussion of the discipline.

Included in each case are questions pertaining to the clinical condition or management of that particular disorder. Selected references are cited after each case for the reader who seeks further information specifically related to the case history. We refer interested readers to standard textbooks of urology for additional insight into the field.

acknowledgments

I would like to thank my dear nurse and secretary, Elizabeth Rosenfeld, without whose untiring and devoted efforts none of my work would be possible. My associate, Dr. Louis J. Rosenfeld, reviewed the manuscript and gave many helpful suggestions. He is a great teacher and physician, and has been a guiding light through my entire professional career. Dr. Harry Newman allowed me the opportunity of preparing this manuscript and has also been a source of inspiration and guidance. Dr. Selwyn Levitt and Dr. John R. Herman were kind enough to allow me to use several of their cases in this presentation.

BF

To Hansi
without whose encouragement
this would not have been possible.

contents

I: URINARY OBSTRUCTION

INTRODUCTION 1

1 : 2-week-old Boy with Diarrhea, Vomiting and Fever . . 3
2 : 43-year-old Male with Frequency, Nocturia and Recurrent UTI 9
3 : 73-year-old Male with Nocturia and Hesitancy 13
4 : 4-month-old Girl with Lower Abdominal Mass 17
5 : 6-1/2-year-old Girl with Flank Pain and Fever . . . 23
6 : Asymptomatic 34-year-Male 27
7 : 2-year-old Child with an Abdominal Mass 36
8 : 32-year-old Male with Difficulty Voiding 40

II: GENITOURINARY INJURY

INTRODUCTION 45

9 : 16-year-old Male with Injury to Left Flank 48
10 : 17-year-old Male with Stab Wounds 55
11 : 11-year-old Boy Hit by Automobile 59
12 : 41-year-old Female with Fever and Urinary Leakage, Posthysterectomy 64
13 : 20-year-old Male with Abdominal Trauma 71
14 : 24-year-old Male with Gunshot Wound 74
15 : 24-year-old Male with Perineal Injury 78
16 : 52-year-old Female with Urinary Leakage After Abdominal Surgery 83
17 : 36-year-old Female with Urinary Leakage Following Hysterectomy 89

III: VESICOURETERAL REFLUX

INTRODUCTION 93

18 : 6-year-old Girl with Urinary Tract Infection 95
19 : 9-year-old Girl with Urinary Tract Infection 100
20 : 2-month-old Child with an Abdominal Mass 105
21 : 67-year-old Male with Gross Hematuria 109

IV: "NONSPECIFIC" INFECTIONS

INTRODUCTION 111

- 22 : 72-year-old Female with Nausea and Vomiting 112
- 23 : 25-year-old Female with Dysuria and Fever 116
- 24 : 27-year-old Male with Right Upper Quadrant Pain . . 120
- 25 : 57-year-old Female with Gross Hematuria 125
- 26 : 64-year-old Male with Frequency, Dysuria and Nocturia 129

V: TUBERCULOSIS

INTRODUCTION 132

- 27 : 32-year-old Male with Frequency, Urgency and Dysuria 134
- 28 : 29-year-old Female with Difficulty in Voiding 138
- 29 : 45-year-old Male with Pyuria 144

VI: RENAL TUMORS

INTRODUCTION 146

- 30 : 69-year-old Male with Hematuria 149
- 31 : 54-year-old Female with Flank Pain and Hematuria . . 155
- 32 : 61-year-old Male with Hematuria 161
- 33 : 53-year-old Female with Abdominal Pain 166
- 34 : 65-year-old Male with Chest Mass 170
- 35 : 8-year-old Boy with an Abdominal Mass 178
- 36 : 40-year-old Male with Right Renal Colic 184
- 37 : 8-month-old Child with Fever, Weight Loss and Sepsis 189
- 38 : 42-year-old Male with Gross Hematuria 191
- 39 : 68-year-old Male with Difficulty Voiding 193

VII: BLADDER TUMORS

INTRODUCTION 199

- 40 : 61-year-old Male with Gross Hematuria 201
- 41 : 52-year-old Male with Gross Hematuria 204

42 : 57-year-old Male with Gross Hematuria 207
43 : 65-year-old Male with Gross Hematuria 209

VIII: CARCINOMA OF THE PROSTATE

INTRODUCTION 213

44 : 62-year-old Male with Difficulty Voiding 215
45 : 58-year-old Male with Frequency 217
46 : 66-year-old Male with Nodule of Prostate 220

IX: RENAL CALCULI

INTRODUCTION 224

47 : 39-year-old Male with Painless Hematuria 226
48 : 41-year-old Male with Renal Colic 229
49 : 65-year-old Female with Hematuria 236
50 : 52-year-old Female with Hematuria and Flank Pain . . 240
51 : 26-year-old Female with Hematuria During
     Pregnancy 246
52 : 65-year-old Male with Dysuria and Frequency 254
53 : 56-year-old Female with Frequency and Dysuria. . . 258

X: THE ADRENAL GLAND

INTRODUCTION 264

54 : 40-year-old Female with Hypertension and
     Amenorrhea 265
55 : 41-year-old Female with Hypertension 269
56 : 79-year-old Female with Nausea, Vomiting and
     Abdominal Mass 272

XI: NEUROGENIC BLADDER

INTRODUCTION 277

57 : 74-year-old Male with Cerebrovascular Accident . . 279
58 : 17-year-old Boy with Neck Injury 284
59 : 48-year-old Male with Fracture of L4 and L5
     Vertebrae and Urinary Tract Infection 289
60 : 34-year-old Male with Difficulty Voiding 294

DIAGNOSES: CASE STUDIES	299
INDEX	305
POST-TEST	308
Answer Key	324

notice

The editor(s) and/or author(s) and the publisher of this book have made every effort to ensure that all therapeutic modalities that are recommended are in accordance with accepted standards at the time of publication.

The drugs specified within this book may not have specific approval by the Food and Drug Administration in regard to the indications and dosages that are recommended by the editor(s) and/or author(s). The manufacturer's package insert is the best source of current prescribing information.

CHAPTER I

URINARY OBSTRUCTION

INTRODUCTION

Obstructive uropathy accounts for the majority of patients seen by the practicing urologist. Uppermost in the urologist's mind is the back pressure effect on the renal parenchyma and its deleterious effect on renal function. The obstructive process can occur anywhere along the course of the collecting system, from the urethral meatus to obstruction of a major calyx, and cause destruction of only a portion of the kidney. The obstructive lesions are generally classified into congenital or acquired types. The more common congenital sites of urinary obstruction are posterior urethral valves in boys, distal urethral obstruction in girls, ureterocele, and ureteropelvic junction obstruction. Examples of acquired obstruction are urethral strictures, bladder neck obstruction secondary to benign prostatic hyperplasia or bladder neck contracture, tuberculous urethral strictures, cancer, or ureteral calculi.

Any pathologic process causing obstruction to the flow of urine, be it by mechanical means or atonic neuromuscular disease, will eventually give rise to hydronephrosis and subsequent renal atrophy. The complicating factors in obstruction are infection and stone formation, both leading to further renal function deterioration.

The pathologic process seen in the bladder consequent to obstruction is similar to that seen in the heart. In order to overcome the increased resistance of the obstructing lesion, the bladder musculature will undergo hypertrophy, thereby increasing the pressure by increasing the strength of contraction, and will compensate to empty itself. As the obstruction progresses and the hypertrophied organ can no longer attain the pressures necessary to empty itself, the bladder will begin to dilate. With this, the hypertrophied muscles will show trabeculae. With progression of this process, the bladder mucosa will protrude through these trabeculae, and cellules will be followed by saccule formation; finally diverticula will form. Larger and larger amounts of residual urine will remain in the bladder. If the obstruction is allowed to proceed unabated, the upper tracts are eventually affected. In a similar manner, the muscles of the ureter become thickened to overcome the distal resistance. With further decompensation, dilation and tortuosity will be seen, and with total decompensation, there will be complete inability to propel the urinary stream along its normal course. In the renal pelvis and calyces, normal pressures are very low, ranging from 0 to 15 mmHg. As the pressure is increased due to distal obstruction, the pelvis and calyces begin to dilate. The early pathologic changes are seen in the area of the calyces where the calyx becomes flattened and then clubbed due to pressure necrosis and absorption of the papilla. When back pressure increases, the tubules become dilated and undergo ischemic atrophy. As more and more renal parenchyma undergo pressure atrophy, renal decompensation will ensue.

Urinary Obstruction

CASE 1: 2-WEEK-OLD BOY WITH DIARRHEA, VOMITING AND FEVER

HISTORY

A 2-week-old, full-term baby boy was admitted with the chief complaint of diarrhea, vomiting, and fever for 2 days. He was found to have an elevated BUN in the range of 28 to 56 mg%. He was in severe electrolyte imbalance with pyuria and sepsis. The initial urine cultures were positive, showing over 100,000 colonies of E. coli per cc. After recovery from acidosis and dehydration, the urologist was consulted for the problem of pyuria.

PHYSICAL EXAMINATION

Examination revealed a pale, weak, fairly well-nourished and developed, full-term baby boy. The abdomen was slightly bulging. The liver and spleen could not be palpated. There were good bowel sounds. The right kidney was palpable and of soft consistency. There were no masses palpable. The external genitalia appeared normal. A poor urinary stream was noted on voiding.

LABORATORY DATA

Hematocrit 38%; WBC 3,200; urinalysis showed 4 to 8 white cells per high power field. Urine culture showed no growth. The electrolytes were normal. BUN 33 mg%, creatinine .9 mg%.

QUESTIONS

1. Differential diagnosis at this point would be:
   A. Ureteropelvic junction obstruction
   B. Posterior urethral valves
   C. Ureterovesical junction obstruction
   D. All of the above
   E. None of the above

2. The first diagnostic procedure to be done would be:
   A. Intravenous urogram
   B. Retrograde pyelogram
   C. Voiding cystourethrogram
   D. Cystopanendoscopy
   E. Bilateral retrogrades

3. Posterior urethral valves are best diagnosed by:
   A. Intravenous urogram
   B. Retrograde cystogram
   C. Voiding cystourethrogram
   D. Cystoscopy

Intravenous urogram (Fig. 1.1) showed bilateral ureterohydronephrosis. Voiding cystourethrogram revealed Grade IV vesicoureteral reflux with evidence of obstruction of the posterior urethra showing typical formation of posterior urethral valves (Fig. 1.2).

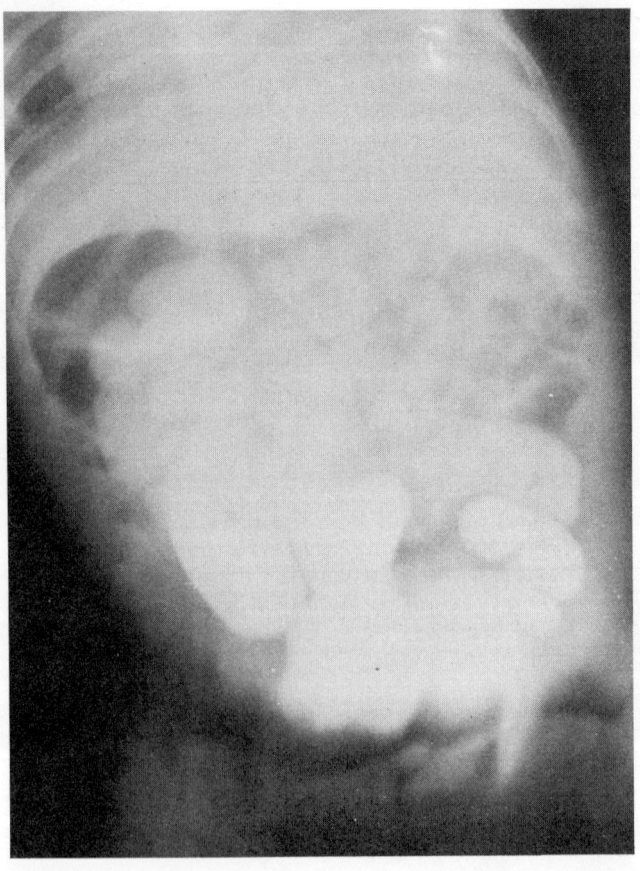

FIG. 1.1: Intravenous urogram showing bilateral ureterohydronephrosis.

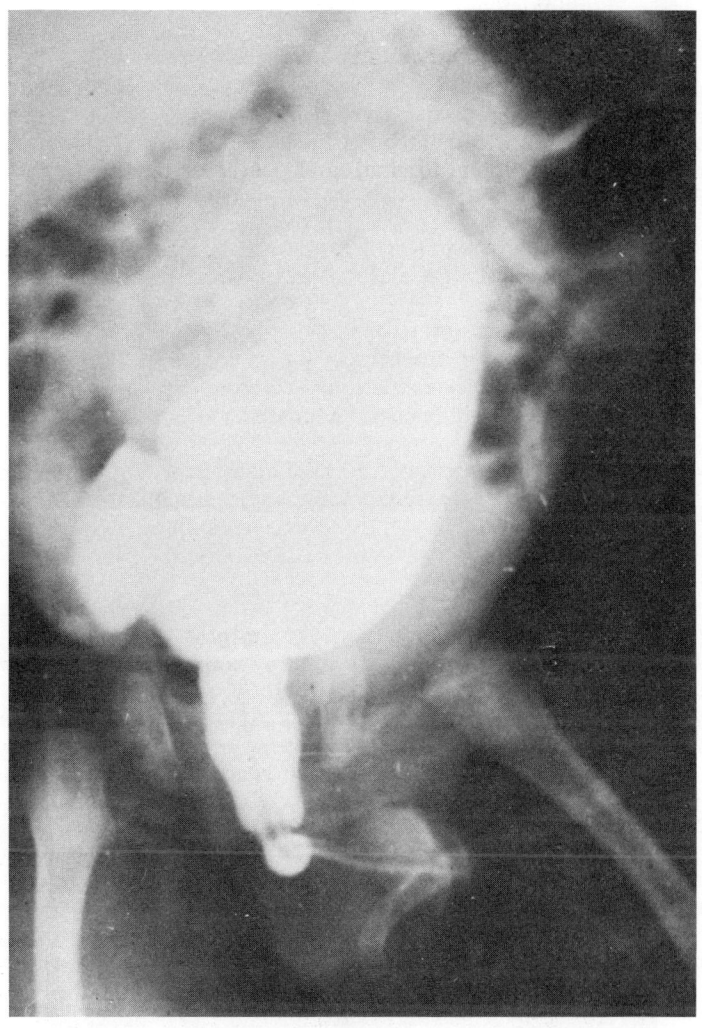

FIG. 1.2: Voiding cystourethrogram showing posterior urethral valves and marked reflux.

4. The most common type of posterior urethral valve is:
   A. Young I
   B. Young II
   C. Young III

5. Patients with urethral valves commonly present:
   A. At birth
   B. By 3 months
   C. By one year
   D. Before puberty
   E. After puberty

6. Patients who present with fever, uremia and sepsis secondary to posterior urethral valves are best handled by:
   A. Nephrostomy
   B. Urethral catheter
   C. Suprapubic cystostomy
   D. Transurethral resection of valves
   E. Tubeless cutaneous ureterostomy

After correction of electrolyte imbalance, dehydration and recovery from sepsis by intensive antibiotic administration, bilateral loop ureteropyelostomies were performed.

CLINICAL COURSE

Postoperative course was benign. Creatinine clearance was 14 cc per minute on each side. Voiding cystourethrograms showed less dilation of both ureters and proximal urethra. Two weeks postoperatively, a transurethral resection of the urethral valves was performed through a perineal urethrostomy. Postoperative course following T.U.R. was also benign. The perineal catheter drained no urine and was discontinued on the first postoperative day. The perineal incision dried and healed promptly. After six months of drainage by loop cutaneous ureterostomy, a repeat cystourethrogram again showed bilateral vesicoureteral reflux, but the valves were seen to be absent. He underwent bilateral ureteral reimplantation for correction of reflux. Repeat voiding cystourethrogram three months following this showed no reflux and a normal urethra. He then underwent closure of both ureterostomies by a staged procedure and has done well since that time. Creatinine remains in the range of 0.9-1.1 mg%.

ANSWERS AND DISCUSSION

1. (D) All of the choices indicated are possibilities in the etiology of this child's urinary tract infection. However, the

Urinary Obstruction

most likely cause in a week-old male would be posterior urethral valves.

2. (A) The initial step in any urologic evaluation would be an intravenous urogram if the renal function permits. This gives us a good idea of the condition of the upper urinary tracts and a clue as to the etiology of obstruction, if any. Upper tract obstruction such as ureteropelvic junction obstruction would be diagnosed in this manner.

3. (C) Demonstration of valves is best seen on voiding cystourethrogram, as in Fig. 1.2. It can be seen that the valve leaflets are descending through the external sphincter giving the typical convex appearance.

4. (A) Type I. There are three types of posterior urethral valves as described by Young. The most common, Type I, are an exaggeration of the normal mucosal folds extending distally from the verumontanum to the external sphincter. In Type II, they extend from the verumontanum to the bladder neck. Type III is an iris type structure either above or below the verumontanum.

5. (C) The majority of cases of valves present before one year of age, about half present prior to 3 months. When they are present at birth, there is a failure to void. Later there is a failure to thrive, distended abdomen, urinary infection, gastrointestinal symptoms, etc.

6. (B) If the child is relatively well and there is no significant azotemia, transurethral resection of the valves would be the preferred form of therapy, even in the presence of markedly dilated upper urinary tracts.

In this case, however, with the presence of sepsis and azotemia, preliminary diversion of the urine is best prior to definitive therapy of the valve. A temporary type of diversion is usually performed. This can be accomplished by any of the methods cited in the question, but most patients will respond to temporary urethral catheter drainage. If Foley catheter drainage combined with antibiotics fails to control the infection, high cutaneous ureterostomy or pyelostomy should be performed, as was done in the case cited.

REFERENCES

1. Hendren WH: Posterior urethral valves in boys: A broad clinical spectrum. J Urol 106:298-307, 1971.

2. Waldbaum RS and Marshal VF: Posterior urethral valves: Evaluation and surgical management. J Urol 103:801-809, 1970.

3. Williams DI: Pediatric Urology, Appleton-Century-Crofts, London, 1968, pp. 254-263.

Urinary Obstruction

CASE 2: 43-YEAR-OLD MALE WITH FREQUENCY, NOCTURIA AND RECURRENT UTI

HISTORY

A 43-year-old man was admitted to the hospital because of urinary frequency, nocturia 2 to 3 times, and recurrent urinary tract infections for many years. There was no history of gross hematuria, back pain, or passage of urinary calculus. He had been treated with multiple antibiotics and chemotherapy without success. Past medical history revealed that he had had epilepsy since 1960, and had had hepatitis in 1964. Bilateral inguinal hernias were repaired in 1966 and 1969.

PHYSICAL EXAMINATION

On admission, BP normal; heart, chest and abdomen were negative. Rectal examination revealed that he had a minimally enlarged prostate which was not tender, smooth and mobile. Seminal vesicles could be palpated. There was no deformity of the spine, no costovertebral angle tenderness.

LABORATORY DATA

Urinalysis showed 12 to 14 WBC per high power field. Urine culture showed over 100,000 colonies of E. coli sensitive to all antibiotics tested. Chemical profile was normal. BUN 13 mg%. I.V. urogram showed normal upper tracts. A retrograde cystogram revealed a large diverticulum of the right side (Fig. 2.1). Postevacuation film with the catheter failed to empty the diverticulum.

QUESTIONS

1. The most likely diagnosis in this case would be:
    A. Carcinoma of prostate
    B. Benign prostatic hypertrophy
    C. Vesical neck contracture
    D. Chronic prostatitis
    E. Chronic pyelonephritis

2. The significance of the diverticulum not emptying on postevacuation film is that:
    A. The catheter is plugged
    B. There is bladder neck obstruction
    C. There is a stone in the diverticulum
    D. There is poor tone to the diverticulum

10/ Case 2 Urinary Obstruction

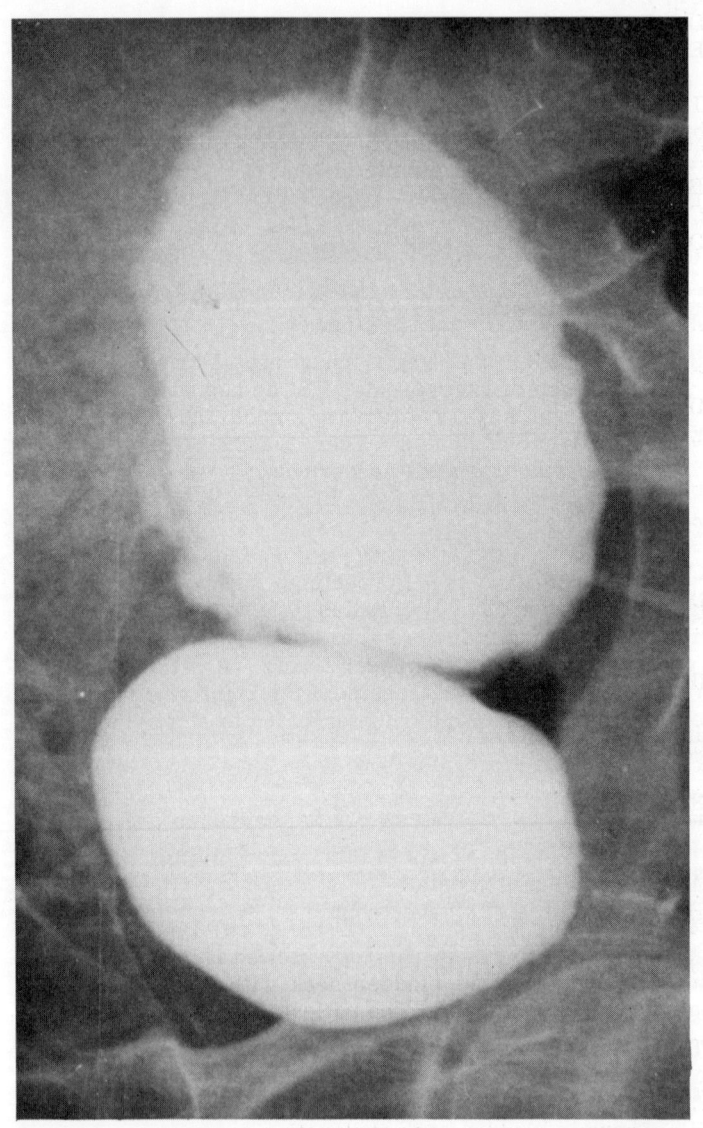

FIG. 2.1: Retrograde cystogram showing large diverticulum on right side of bladder.

Urinary Obstruction

3. The proper therapy for this patient is:
   A. Transurethral resection
   B. Y-V plasty of the bladder neck
   C. Diverticulectomy
   D. B & C
   E. None of the above

4. The diagnosis of vesical neck contracture is best confirmed by:
   A. Rectal examination
   B. Intravenous urogram
   C. Voiding cystourethrogram
   D. Panendoscopy

5. Diverticulum is differentiated from bladder in cystogram by:
   A. Diverticulum is always smaller
   B. Diverticulum is always larger
   C. Diverticulum is smooth
   D. Diverticulum is "scalloped"
   E. None of the above

6. Indications for surgery in a diverticulum of the bladder are:
   A. Size
   B. Failure to empty
   C. Infection
   D. All of the above
   E. None of the above

CLINICAL COURSE

The urinary stream was observed and was fair. Residual urine was 175cc. Cystometrogram showed the first urge to void at 350cc and a bladder capacity of 500cc. The maximum voluntary voiding pressure was 90mm with normal sensation and reflexes. This represented a normal cystometric curve; however, the voiding pressure was markedly elevated. Cystoscopy showed mildly trabeculated bladder, with an opening of a diverticulum 1 cm in diameter at the lateral wall and about 1 cm above the right ureteral orifice. Panendoscopy showed a high bladder neck with a small opening of the bladder neck with a fairly normal prostate and verumontanum. The patient underwent a diverticulectomy and Y-V plasty of the bladder neck. His postoperative course was uneventful; three months later, he was voiding with no nocturia, and the urine was sterile without antibiotics.

12/ Case 2   Urinary Obstruction

ANSWERS AND DISCUSSION

1. (C) With a long history of urinary tract infection in a 43-year-old male, the most likely cause would be recurrent prostatitis with resultant vesical neck contracture. Carcinoma of the prostate and benign prostatic hypertrophy would be likely with the findings of a minimally enlarged prostate that is smooth, mobile and nontender. He evidently has, or has had, chronic prostatitis, but there must be an element of obstruction present in the face of a bladder diverticulum. A diagnosis of chronic pyelonephritis cannot be made on the basis of the information given here.

2. (D) D is the best answer here. A diverticulum of the bladder is an outpouching of the bladder mucosa through the trabeculated muscle layer, secondary to long-standing obstruction. The significance of not emptying on a postevacuation film with a catheter in place makes one deduce that, if the bladder neck obstruction alone were corrected, the diverticulum would continue to carry a residual urine with resultant stasis and infection.

3. (D) Because of the above, diverticulectomy, accompanied by some procedure to alleviate the bladder neck obstruction, would be the procedure of choice for this patient. Transurethral resection alone would not help since the diverticulum would not empty with this alone.

4. (D) On panendoscopy of the urethra, there is difficulty in engaging the panendoscope through the vesical neck. It is notoriously difficult to diagnose vesical neck contracture on the basis of voiding cystourethrogram.

5. (C) A diverticulum of the bladder is an out-pouching of mucosa through the trabeculated muscle of the bladder wall, as shown in Fig. 2.1. Therefore, a diverticulum will always look smooth on cystography, while the bladder will be trabeculated.

6. (D) The best answer is B, although all can be a good indication. In cystography, the bladder is generally emptied through the urethral catheter and, if contrast material remains in the diverticulum, this is an indication that it will not empty when relief of the bladder neck obstruction is carried out.

CASE 3: 73-YEAR-OLD MALE WITH NOCTURIA AND HESITANCY

HISTORY

A 73-year-old male was seen because of urinary frequency, nocturia 4 to 6 times, and hesitancy and decrease in force of his urinary stream. There was no history of urinary tract infections, flank pain, fever or hematuria. He had bronchiectasis for many years, but was on no particular treatment for this at the time he was seen. Past medical history was otherwise negative.

PHYSICAL EXAMINATION

Examination revealed a well-developed, well-nourished male in no distress. Vital signs were normal. Chest was clear to percussion and auscultation. Abdominal examination was normal. On rectal examination, the prostate was massively enlarged and nontender. Remainder of the physical was within normal limits.

LABORATORY DATA

Urinalysis, hemogram, BUN, electrolytes, acid phosphatase and urine culture were all within normal limits. Intravenous urogram showed prompt bilateral excretion with normal upper tracts. The excretory cystogram showed a large intravesical prostate (Fig. 3.1). Cystoscopy revealed a markedly trabeculated bladder with no stone or tumor.

CLINICAL COURSE

A retropubic prostatectomy was performed and the patient made an uneventful recovery. Two months following surgery, he was virtually free of any urologic symptoms and the urine was sterile.

QUESTIONS

1. Benign enlargement of the prostate is most commonly found in the:
    A. Lateral lobes
    B. Middle lobe
    C. Subcervical lobe
    D. Anterior lobes
    E. Posterior lobe

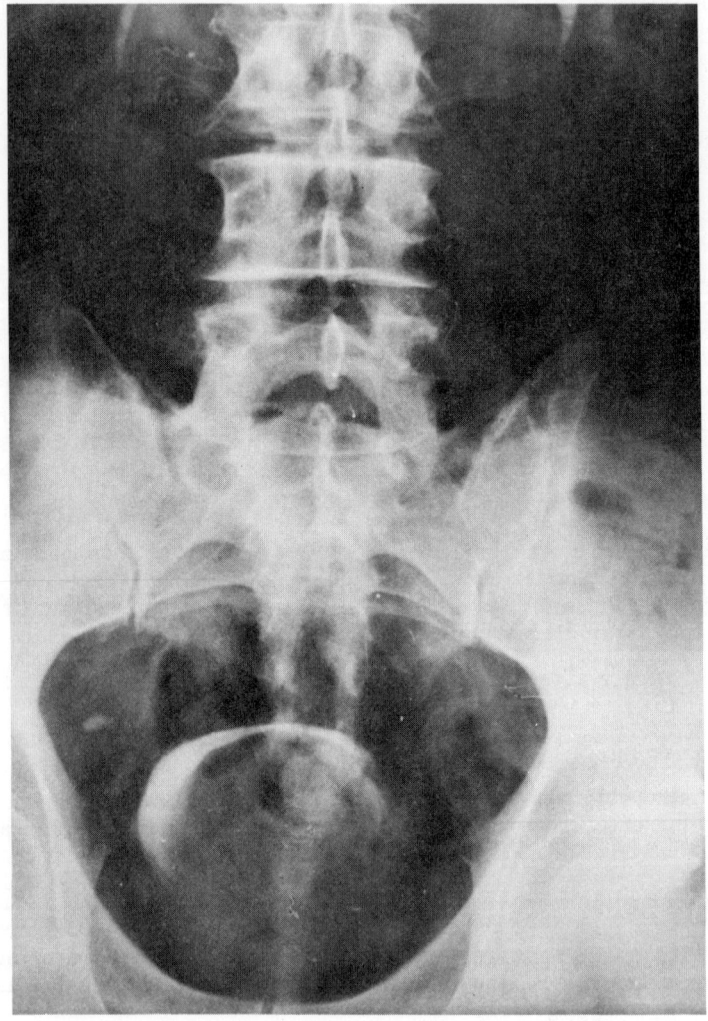

FIG. 3.1: Intravenous urogram showing a very large intravesical prostate pushing the base of the bladder superiorly.

Urinary Obstruction

2. Carcinoma of the prostate is most commonly found in the:
   A. Lateral lobes
   B. Middle lobe
   C. Subcervical lobe
   D. Anterior lobe
   E. Posterior lobe

3. Treatment of benign prostatic hypertrophy is best carried out by:
   A. Transurethral resection
   B. Suprapubic approach
   C. Retropubic approach
   D. Perineal approach
   E. All of the above

4. The best indication for surgery for benign prostatic hypertrophy is:
   A. The size of the gland
   B. Frequency of urination
   C. Severe dysuria
   D. Residual urine greater than 100cc
   E. Nocturia 4-5 times

(T)RUE OR (F)ALSE:

5. Following prostatectomy for benign hypertrophy, the development of carcinoma is rare.

6. Benign prostatic hypertrophy has been shown to respond to the administration of progestational agents.

7. The earliest symptom of prostatic obstruction is frequency of urination.

ANSWERS AND DISCUSSION

1. (A) Three lobes commonly undergo hyperplasia, but the lateral lobes are the more common. The gland becomes elongated and enlarges either toward the rectum or toward the bladder neck, thus causing the intravesical protrusion as seen in Fig. 3.1.

2. (E) Most malignancies originate in the posterior lobe of the prostate in the surgical capsule and can often coexist with benign enlargement or develop after removal of benign prostatic hyperplasia. Occasionally, a "focus" of carcinoma is found within the hyperplastic benign prostatic nodules.

3. (E) Treatment can be by open surgery or transurethral resection. In general, glands smaller than 40 gm are treated by transurethral resection, while those larger than 40 gm are treated by open prostatectomy. The various approaches used in open prostatectomy are the suprapubic, retropubic, and perineal. Each has its own advantages and disadvantages, the choice being the one most familiar to the operating surgeon.

4. (D) Criteria for operation vary among surgeons, but the <u>best</u> indication for surgery would be an increase in residual urine. The other symptoms and signs mentioned can be due to other causes; and, before surgery is contemplated, definite obstruction would have to be demonstrated. The size of the gland alone is not a good indication for surgery; very small glands sometimes cause marked obstruction and very large glands, at times, cause no obstruction at all.

5. (F) As stated in answer No. 2, the incidence of carcinoma of the prostate after surgery for benign disease is identical to that without the operation.

6. (T) There is a great deal of literature showing decrease in symptoms as well as the size of the prostate resulting from the administration of delalutin, cyproterone acetate, as well as other progestational agents. This remains investigative at this time and is not in wide use.

7. (F) The first symptom the patient usually notices with prostatic obstruction is slowing of the urinary stream.

REFERENCES

1. Millin T, McCalister, CLO and Kelly PM: Retropubic prostatectomy. Lancet 1:381-385, 1947.

2. Hudson PB and Stout AP: An Atlas of Prostatic Surgery. W. B. Saunders Co., Philadelphia, 1962.

3. Scott WW and Wade JC: Medical treatment of benign nodular prostatic hyperplasia with cyproterone acetate. J Urol 101:81-85, 1969.

4. Geller J, Angist A, Nako K, and Newman A: Therapy with progestational agents for advanced benign prostatic hyperplasia. JAMA 210:1421-1427, 1969.

Urinary Obstruction   Case 4/ 17

CASE 4: 4-MONTH-OLD GIRL WITH LOWER ABDOMINAL MASS

HISTORY

A 4-month-old baby girl was admitted to the hospital because of a lower abdominal mass. Two weeks prior to admission, she had had diarrhea which was treated with Lomotil. The child was voiding until the evening before admission and then had stopped. There was no history of urinary difficulty prior to this. The diarrhea stopped on the day of admission, but the appetite was poor.

PHYSICAL EXAMINATION

Examination revealed a temperature of 100.8°; the heart rate was 140 per minute; respirations were 70 per minute. She was noted to be an acutely ill, tachypneic and pale infant. Examination of the abdomen revealed a distended bladder. There were no other masses. The remainder of the physical examination was within normal limits. Catheterization of the bladder yielded 150cc of cloudy urine.

LABORATORY DATA

Revealed hematocrit and hemoglobin normal. WBC 11,700 with a shift to the left. Urine showed many RBC's and WBC's with 2+ albumin. BUN 71 mg%. Blood gases revealed a pH of 7.43 and a PCO_2 of 24. Sodium and chlorides were normal. CO_2 was 5 mEq/l. Potassium 6.1 mEq/l.

QUESTIONS

1. The differential diagnosis in this child would include which of the following?
    A. Urethral stricture
    B. Ectopic ureterocele
    C. Bladder neck contracture
    D. Posterior urethral valves
    E. All of the above

2. The most likely diagnosis would be:
    A. Urethral stricture
    B. Ectopic ureterocele
    C. Bladder neck contracture
    D. Posterior urethral valves

3. The above diagnosis can best be made by:
   A. Intravenous pyelogram
   B. Retrograde cystogram
   C. Cystoscopy
   D. Urethroscopy

4. The ectopic ureterocele is usually found in:
   A. The upper segment of a duplex kidney
   B. The lower segment of a duplex kidney
   C. An ectopic kidney
   D. A solitary kidney

5. The most common cause of urinary retention for little girls is:
   A. Urethral stricture
   B. Bladder neck obstruction
   C. Ectopic ureterocele
   D. Psychogenic

6. The best treatment of ectopic ureterocele is:
   A. Transurethral resection of the ureterocele with unroofing
   B. Heminephrectomy of the upper segment with reimplantation of the lower segment
   C. Total nephrectomy
   D. Observation
   E. Open bladder with uncapping of ureterocele

7. The most significant abnormality associated with duplicated kidney is:
   A. Renal cysts
   B. Ureterocele
   C. Cystitis
   D. Urethral diverticula
   E. Urethral stricture

CLINICAL COURSE

The child was treated with intravenous fluids, electrolyte replacement and catheter drainage. The BUN dropped to 16 mg% and the electrolytes were corrected. Urine culture showed over 100,000 colonies of Proteus sensitive to ampicillin, which was administered. Her clinical condition improved rapidly with decreased tachypnea, and good hydration and urine output. An intravenous urogram (Fig. 4.1) showed a double-collecting system on the left side of the bladder consistent with ureterocele. Voiding cystourethrogram showed a smooth wall bladder with evidence of reflux into the lower segment on the left side (Fig. 4.2).

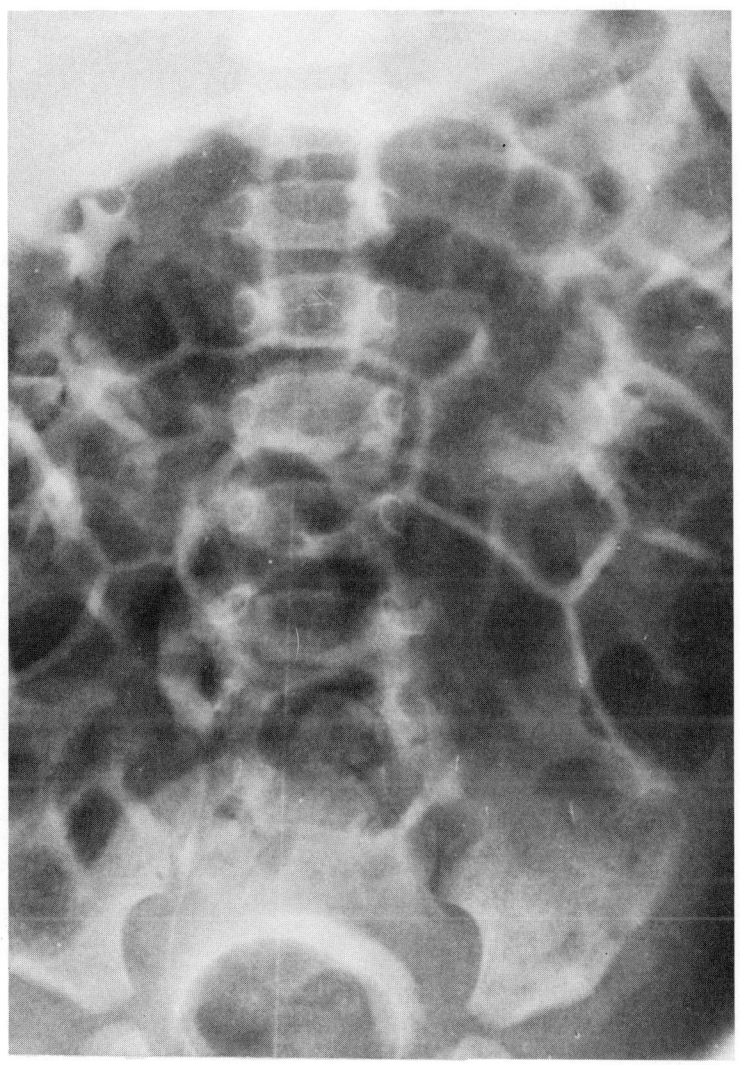

FIG. 4.1: Intravenous urogram showing a double-collecting system on the left, with nonvisualization of the dilated upper segment, and compression of the lower segment downwards. (Note the large filling defect in the bladder indicative of a large ureterocele.)

20/ Case 4 Urinary Obstruction

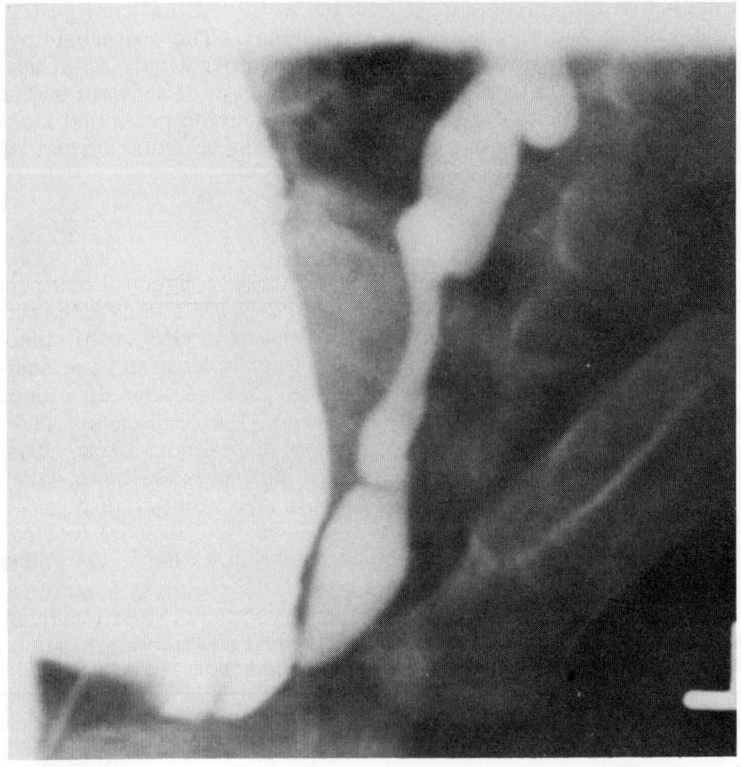

FIG. 4.2: Voiding cystourethrogram showing reflux into the lower ureteral segment on the left.

Urinary Obstruction

Cystoscopy confirmed the presence of the ureterocele. She was taken to the operating room where excision of the ureterocele and left ureteral reimplantation of the lower segment were performed, with the upper left renal segment ureter brought out as a cutaneous ureterostomy. A cystostomy and ureteral splinting catheters were left in place. She had an unremarkable postoperative course. All splints and the cystostomy tube were removed by the 10th postoperative day. Her urine remained uninfected on ampicillin and she voided well. At that time, BUN was 6 mg%, and electrolytes were normal. The ureterostomy never excreted urine, and one month postoperatively a left upper heminephroureterectomy was performed. She again had an unremarkable postoperative course. The urine remained sterile. All chemistries were normal when she was discharged 10 days after her 2nd procedure.

DISCUSSION

This case is an example of a fairly common congenital obstructive lesion namely, ureterocele. This is a ballooning of the submucosal ureter into the bladder, secondary to congenital stenosis of the ureter at its vesical end. Its complications are basically those of obstruction and infection. Stones often develop in these cyst-like masses. If large enough, they can cause bladder neck obstruction by impingement at the bladder neck. They are usually seen in little girls and, as illustrated here, are formed in the upper segment of a duplicated kidney. If possible, ureteral reimplantation with preservation of renal function is the preferred method of management, but as here, very often the renal segment supplying this portion of ureter is destroyed by hydronephrotic changes and must be removed. Heminephrectomy is commonly performed at the time of reimplantation rather than as a secondary procedure in this case.

ANSWERS AND DISCUSSION

1. (E) Any of the answers are a possibility. However, posterior urethral valves almost never occur in little girls, urethral stricture very rarely causes urinary retention, and vesical neck contracture is a very rare disorder in children.

2. (B) See above. Rarely, as in this case, is a ureterocele so large that it causes obstruction of the bladder neck.

3. (A) The filling defect in the bladder seen on intravenous urogram is the characteristic sign of ureterocele especially in the presence of renal duplication. A retrograde cystogram

would show this as well if the contrast were dilute enough. The ureterocele could also be seen by cystourethroscopy.

4. (A) The ectopic ureterocele is almost always borne in the upper pole of a duplex kidney. Females predominate about 7:1. Single ureters are rarely encountered in male cases. The renal element involved is generally small, irregular and dysplastic, but the ureter itself may be dilated and tortuous.

5. (C) The ureterocele may obstruct the bladder neck, causing urinary retention; it is probably the most common cause of retention in infant girls. At times the ureterocele can prolapse through the urethra and present at the meatus.

6. (B) Uncapping of the ureterocele either by the transurethral route or through the open bladder is not an accepted method of management since it leaves a markedly dilated upper segment, with reflux which leads to recurrent infection. The standard treatment is heminephrectomy and total ureterectomy of the upper segment with reimplantation of the lower segment.

7. (B) Ureterocele is the most common condition associated with duplicated collecting system.

REFERENCES

1. Williams DI: Pediatric Urology, Appleton-Century-Crofts, London, 1968, pp. 205-211.

2. Timothy RP, Decter A, and Perlmutter AD: Ureteral duplication: Clinical findings and therapy in 46 children. J Urol 105:445, 1971.

3. Lundin E and Riggs W: Upper urinary tract duplication associated with ectopic ureterocele in childhood and infancy. Acta Radiol 7:13-24, 1968.

4. Johnston JH and Johnson LM: Experience with ectopic ureteroceles. Brit J Urol 41:61-70, 1969.

5. Williams DL and Royle M: Ectopic ureter in the male child. Brit J Urol 41:421-427, 1969.

Urinary Obstruction

CASE 5: 6½-YEAR-OLD GIRL WITH FLANK PAIN AND FEVER

HISTORY

A 6½-year-old female child was well until one day prior to admission when she developed right flank pain, fever, and cloudy urine. She had one previous episode of urinary tract infection 2 years prior to admission which was treated by her family physician with prompt resolution. Past medical history: the child had pneumonia at age 2 and had a T & A at age 4.

PHYSICAL EXAMINATION

Temperature on admission was 102.8; there was voluntary guarding in the right upper and right lower quadrant with rebound and no rigidity. There was right costovertebral angle tenderness.

LABORATORY DATA

WBC 15,900 with a shift to the left. Hematocrit, BUN, FBS, electrolytes: normal. Urinalysis showed many WBC's per high power field. Urine culture grew out 10^5 colonies of E. coli per cc which were sensitive to most antibiotics tested.

QUESTIONS

1. Differential diagnosis from above should include:
   A. Ureteropelvic junction obstruction
   B. Ureteral calculus
   C. Acute pyelonephritis
   D. Renal duplication with hydronephrosis or reflux
   E. All of the above

2. Diagnosis can best be made by:
   A. Intravenous pyelogram
   B. Retrograde cystogram
   C. Voiding cystourethrogram
   D. Cystoscopy

3. Initial therapy should consist of:
   A. Antibiotic therapy
   B. Passage of urethral catheter
   C. Passage of ureteral catheter
   D. Nephrostomy
   E. All of the above

CLINICAL COURSE

Patient was treated with Gantrisin but responded slowly and her temperature gradually came down. I.V. urogram showed a normal left collecting system. There was evidence of double-collecting system on the right and compression of the lower segment (Fig. 5.1). Cystoscopy and panendoscopy were normal. Following this, the patient underwent a right heminephrectomy through a flank incision, the upper segment of the right kidney being removed with the upper portion of ureter. The distal segment of ureter was brought to the skin at this time. One week subsequent to this, through a low abdominal incision, the distal portion of ureter was removed and this was seen to enter the posterior portion of the urethra with complete obstruction at this point. She had a completely benign postoperative course and was discharged on the 8th postoperative day, following the 2nd procedure, at which time her urine was sterile. She has done well since that time and her urine remained sterile.

(T)RUE OR (F)ALSE:

4. Complete duplication of the ureter is a very rare anomaly.

ANSWERS AND DISCUSSION

1. (E) All the conditions mentioned should enter the differential diagnosis from the information available up to this point. The signs and symptoms pointing to the right flank accompanied by the positive urine culture should include all of these diagnoses.

2. (A) Intravenous urogram would best differentiate the above conditions. Ureteropelvic junction obstruction would easily be seen. Ureteral calculi do occur in children but are rare. Renal duplication should always be thought of in cases like this even if the excretory urogram appears normal; a clue to this is sometimes seen with deviation of the midureter caused by a dilated upper segment causing shifting of the visualized segment laterally.

3. (A) Antibiotic therapy should always be given initially prior to any attempt at surgical intervention especially in the untreated child. This often will be successful in decreasing the temperature. One is then able to deal with a child who is less ill and, therefore, there is less of a risk for surgical intervention. Of course, if antibiotic therapy alone fails, some form of drainage would be necessary in an obstructed kidney.

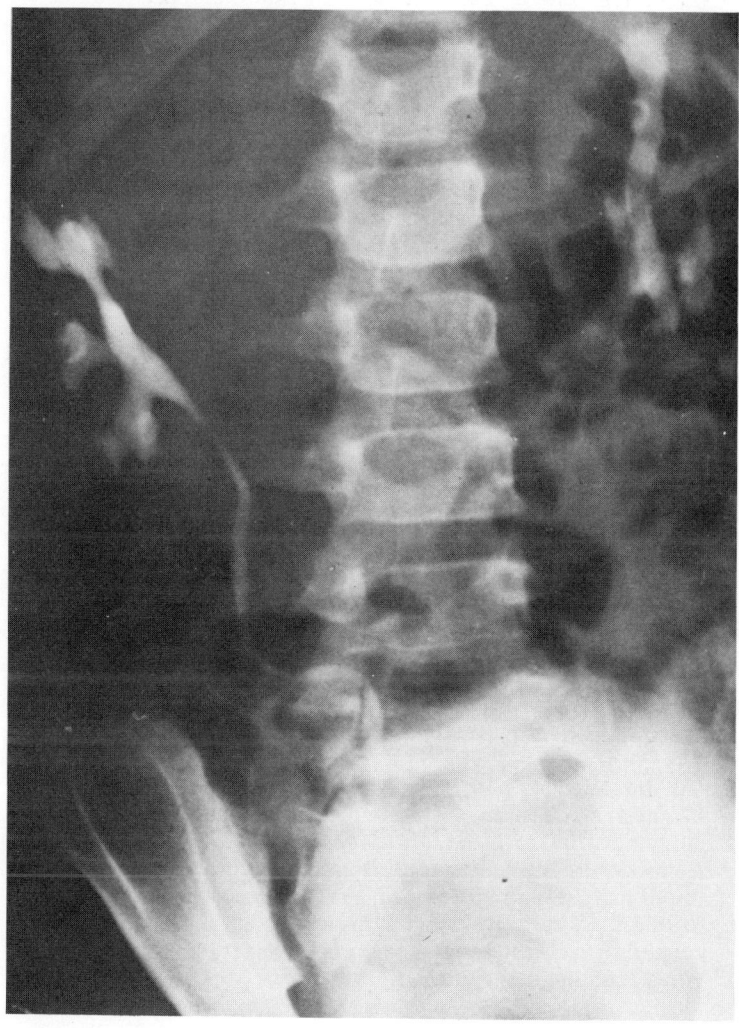

FIG. 5.1: Intravenous urogram with double-collecting system on the right and evidence of compression of the lower segment downward by the hydronephrotic (nonvisualized) upper segment.

4. (F) Duplication of the kidney is a fairly common finding. This may involve only the renal pelvis or part or all of the ureter on one or both sides. In complete duplication of the ureter, the orifice from the upper pelvis is located distal and medial to the one from the lower pelvis. Not uncommonly, the ectopic ureteral orifice can lie extravesically. In the female, this is usually in the vagina and causes incontinence. In the male, the ectopic opening can be in the seminal vesicles or posterior urethra. As in the case depicted, disease is frequently limited to one of the duplicated portions of the kidney and can easily be missed since urographic studies show only the normal portion of the kidney. The upper segment of the kidney is more predisposed to disease, either by ureterocele (Case #4) or congenital stenosis (Case #5) or reflux. Duplication should always be considered when the visualized kidney does not have its full complement of calyces and the pelvis and calyces do not correspond to the size of the renal shadow (Figs. 4.1 and 5.1). When renal damage is not severe, ureteral reimplantation into the bladder is the treatment of choice. When renal damage is marked, as in the previous two cases, partial nephrectomy is necessary.

REFERENCES

1. Amar AD: Lateral ureteral displacement sign of nonvisualized duplication. J Urol 105:638-641, 1971.

2. Timothy RP, Decter A, and Perlmutter AD: Ureteral duplication: Clinical findings and therapy in 46 children. J Urol 105:445, 1971.

Urinary Obstruction

CASE 6: ASYMPTOMATIC 34-YEAR-OLD MALE

HISTORY

A 34-year-old white male was first seen in October 1967. He had a history of passing several calculi, and had been followed for a known calculus in the lower calyx of the left kidney. An intravenous urogram in October 1966, revealed the calculus in the lower pole of the left kidney, and showed fullness of the right renal pelvis, but good cupping of all the calyces (Fig. 6.1). A routine intravenous urogram, repeated in October 1967, revealed marked hydronephrosis on the right with dilation of all the calyces (Fig. 6.2). Patient remained asymptomatic throughout this time. A retrograde ureteropyelogram was performed and showed a normal ureter with obstruction of the right ureteropelvic junction (Fig. 6.3). A 1-hour delayed film following retrograde injection showed marked dilatation of all calyces (Fig. 6.4).

PHYSICAL EXAMINATION

On admission, BP 180/100; the remainder of the physical examination was entirely within normal limits.

CLINICAL COURSE

The kidney was explored through a right flank incision, and the obstruction was found to be secondary to a vessel crossing the ureteropelvic junction. The vessel was freed from this area, and the pelvis promptly emptied. In spite of this, it was elected to perform dismembered pyeloplasty, because of the probability of intrinsic obstruction as well (Fig. 6.5). This was performed without splints or nephrostomy. His postoperative course was uneventful, except for persistent hypertension. A repeat urogram in August 1968, showed good cupping of all calyces, some pyelectasis, and visualization of the lower ureter on a 15-minute film (Fig. 6.6). He continues to do well, and his pyelogram remains normal.

QUESTIONS

1. Ureteropelvic junction obstruction is caused by:
    A. Extrinsic scar formation
    B. Adynamic pelvis
    C. Mucosal valve at ureteropelvic junction
    D. Renal vessel crossing the ureteropelvic junction
    E. All of the above

28/ Case 6 Urinary Obstruction

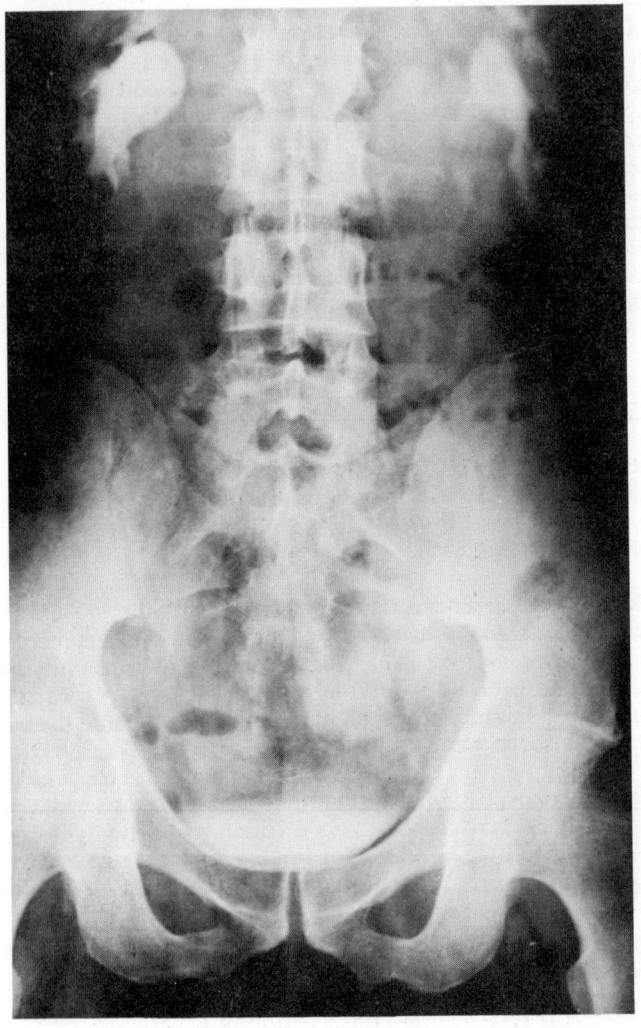

FIG. 6.1: Intravenous urogram, October 1966.

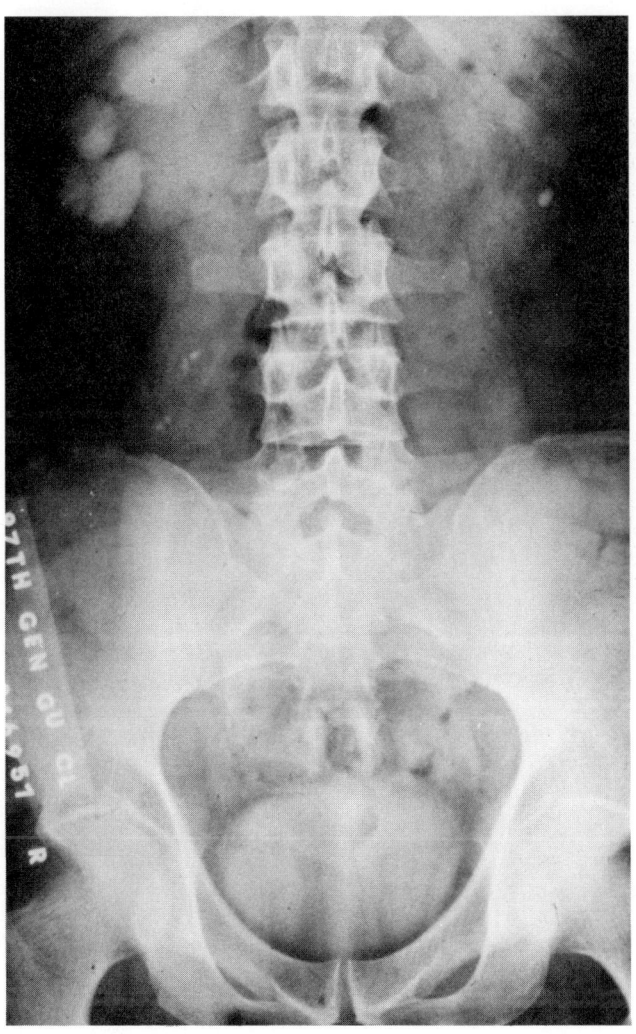

FIG. 6.2: Intravenous urogram, October 1967.

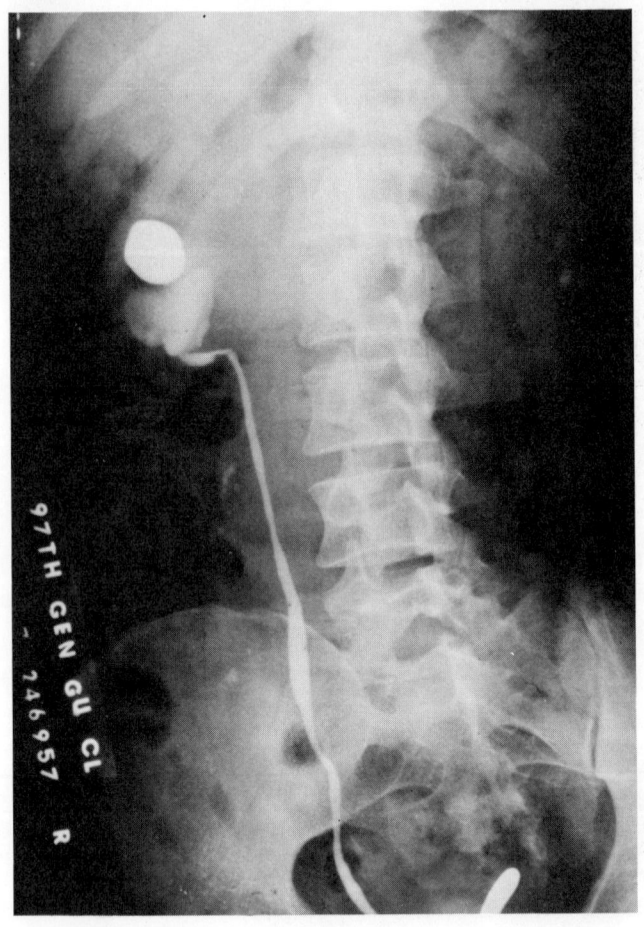

FIG. 6.3: Retrograde ureteropyelogram.

Urinary Obstruction

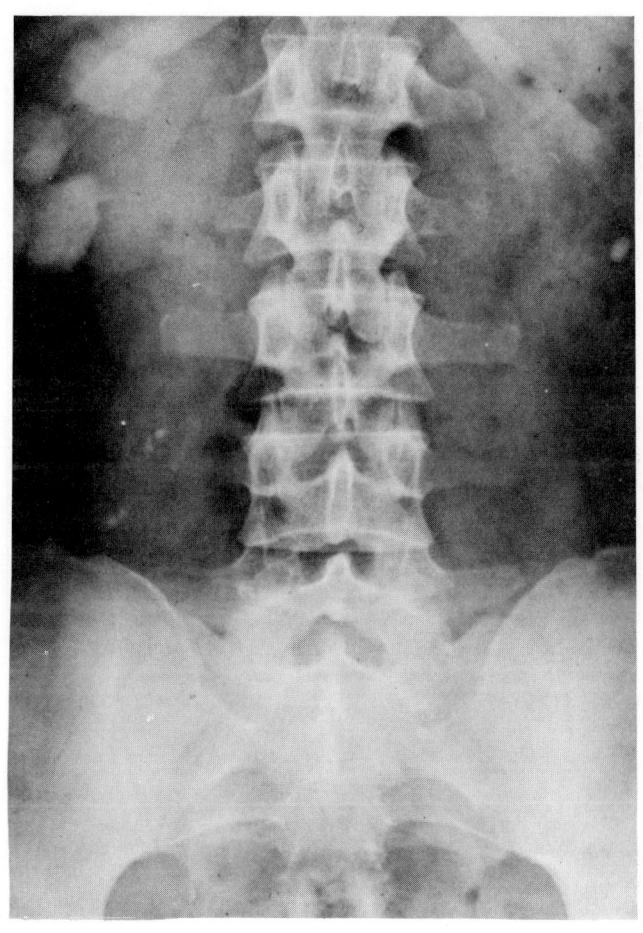

FIG. 6.4: One-hour delayed film of retrograde pyelogram.

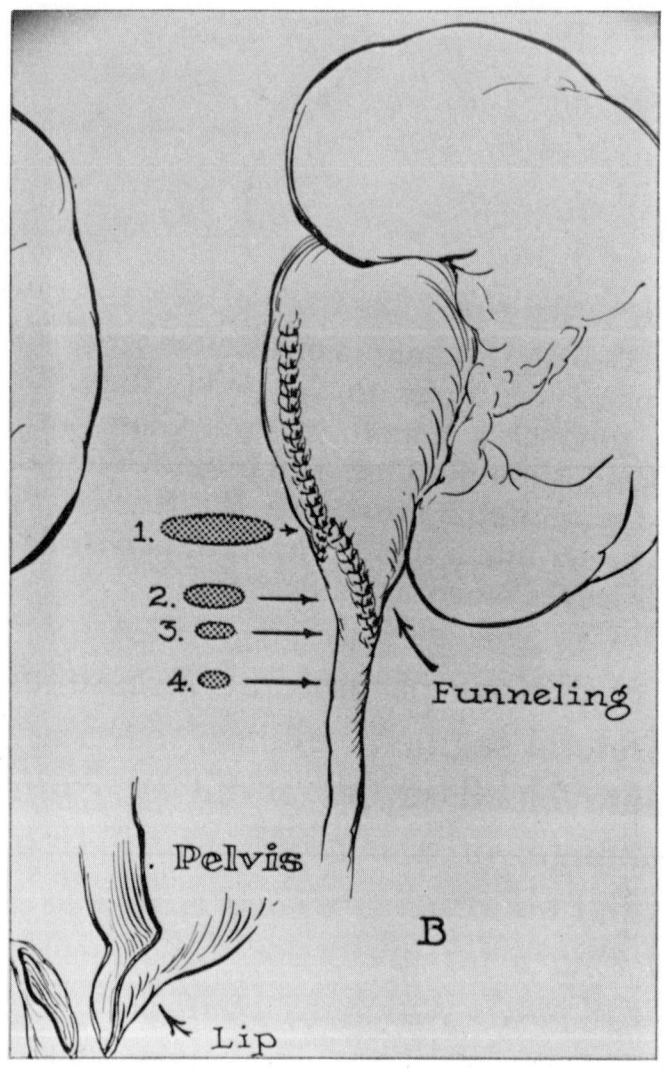

FIG. 6.5: Dismembered pyeloplasty. (From Campbell MF: Urology, W. B. Saunders Co., Philadelphia, 1964.)

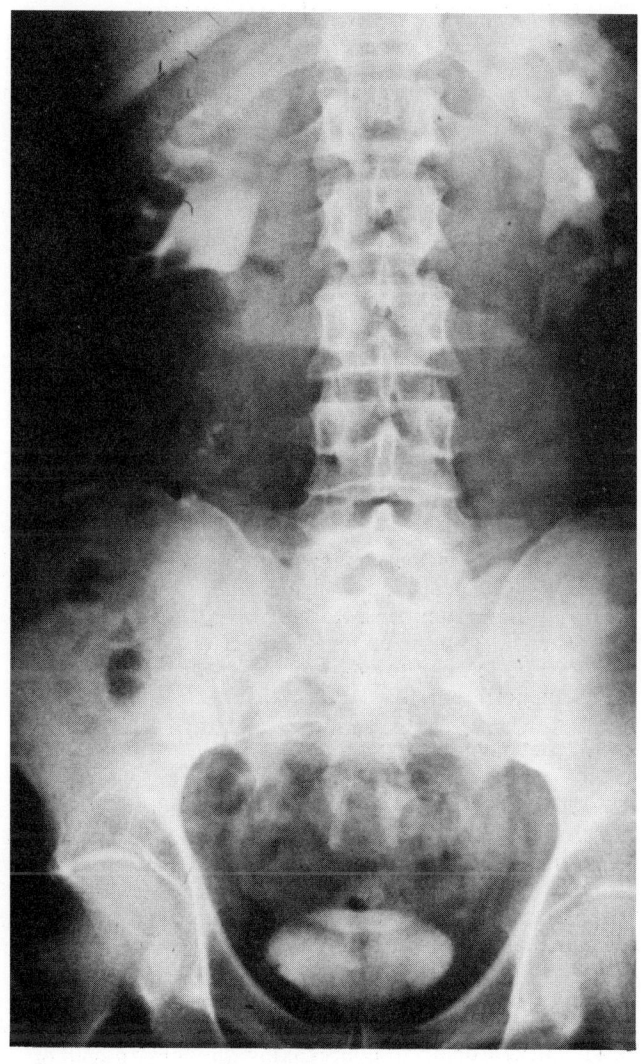

FIG. 6.6: Postoperative intravenous pyelogram.

2. Retrograde pyelography is indicated in this case to:
   A. Demonstrate the point of obstruction
   B. Obtain urine culture from the kidney
   C. Better visualize the collecting system
   D. Rule out other causes of dysfunction

3. Indications for surgery in ureteropelvic junction obstruction include:
   A. Infection
   B. Stone formation
   C. Pain
   D. Hematuria
   E. All of the above

4. Obstruction caused by a vessel crossing the ureteropelvic junction is best treated by:
   A. Freeing of artery and attaching it to an area above the UPJ
   B. Freeing of vessel combined with pyeloplasty
   C. Pyeloplasty alone and bringing vessels anterior to pelvis
   D. Nephrectomy

5. Y-V plasty should be reserved exclusively for:
   A. Vessel at ureteropelvic junction
   B. High insertion of ureter
   C. Mucosal valve causing obstruction
   D. Extrinsic scar formation
   E. Adynamic pelvis

ANSWERS AND DISCUSSIONS

1. (E) Obstruction at the ureteropelvic junction is often an intrinsic, ill-defined lesion described as a mucosal fold obstructing this area. Extrinsic scar formation of unknown etiology occurs in a significant number of patients. Renal vessels crossing the ureteropelvic junction are very often found in these cases, rarely the primary cause of obstruction.

2. (A) In this case, the pelvis was never really completely seen, nor was the ureter visualized. A normal ureter should be visualized prior to undertaking surgery in any of these cases. In this situation, an acorn or bulb-type catheter is placed at the ureteral meatus to visualize the entire ureter. This assures that the obstruction is at the ureteropelvic junction, and not elsewhere along the ureter. In most circumstances, the most convenient and safest time for retrograde

Urinary Obstruction

pyelography is immediately prior to surgical intervention. This insures immediate drainage of the obstructed kidney.

3. (E) Surgical intervention is indicated when there is evidence of progressive or symptomatic disease, such as infection, calculus formation or pain even into late middle age. Unfortunately, indications in this disease process are not exact, and there are no hard and fast rules to go by.

    Pyeloplasty is not always the most conservative surgery. If it can be shown preoperatively by isotope studies, angiography, etc., that there is minimal function and renal tissue present, and one finds only a shell of kidney at the time of surgery - in the presence of a normal contralateral kidney - nephrectomy may be the most prudent course. Certainly, in patients of advanced age, no treatment, or nephrectomy, is often best.

4. (B) Crossing vessels are very rarely the only cause of ureteropelvic junction obstruction, and freeing them only will result in disappointing results in a significant number of cases. It is, therefore, wise to combine freeing of the vessels with some form of pyeloplasty.

5. (B) Foley's Y-V plasty for ureteropelvic junction obstruction is best reserved for high insertion of the ureter into the pelvis. A "V"-shaped incision is made in the pelvis on its anterior and posterior surface, and is extended onto the ureter on its lateral border as a Y incision. The tip of the V is then sutured into the distalmost point in the Y, thus widening the ureteropelvic junction.

REFERENCE

1. Smart WR: Surgical correction of hydronephrosis. In: Campbell MF and Harrison JH: Urology, Volume 3, W.B. Saunders Co., Philadelphia, 1970, p. 2198.

See Case 7 for additional references.

CASE 7: 2-YEAR-OLD CHILD WITH AN ABDOMINAL MASS

HISTORY

A 2-year-old child was referred to the urologist because of a left-sided abdominal mass found by the pediatrician on a routine physical examination. There was no hematuria.

PHYSICAL EXAMINATION

On examination, there was protuberance of the abdomen, and a mass was palpated in the left side which was smooth and extremely firm.

LABORATORY DATA

Routine laboratory studies were normal. An intravenous urogram revealed nonvisualization of the left kidney and a normal right kidney. A left retrograde ureteropyelogram (Fig. 7.1) showed a massive hydronephrotic kidney secondary to a ureteropelvic junction obstruction. Renal scan and renogram failed to reveal uptake of isotope.

CLINICAL COURSE

The kidney was explored the following day, and a massive hydronephrosis was found with just a shell of renal parenchyma. Nephrectomy was performed, and the child made an uneventful recovery.

QUESTIONS

1. The following are causes of abdominal masses in children:
   A. Wilms' tumor
   B. Neuroblostoma
   C. Hydronephrosis
   D. Infantile polycystic kidneys
   E. All of the above

2. Hydronephrosis can be differentiated from neoplasm of the kidney by:
   A. Transillumination
   B. Firmness of the mass
   C. Irregularity of the mass
   D. Extension of mass across midline
   E. All of the above

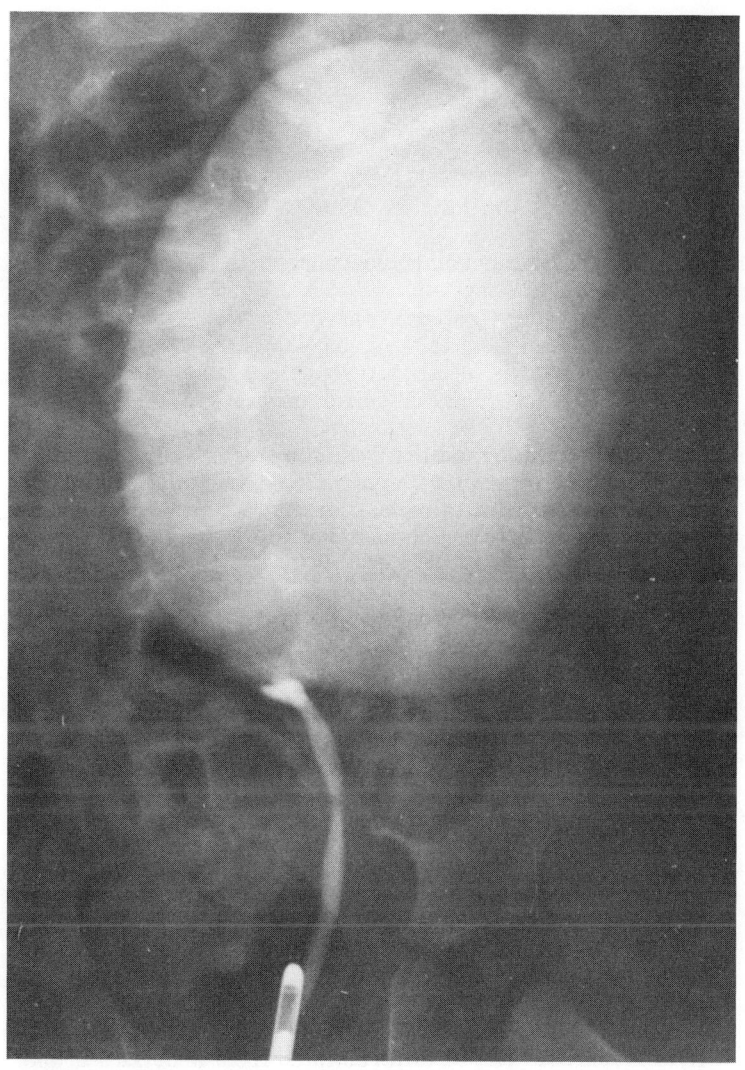

FIG. 7.1: Retrograde pyelogram showing ureteropelvic junction obstruction and massive hydronephrosis.

3. Bilateral ureteropelvic obstruction occurs in approximately:
   A. 5% of cases
   B. 10% of cases
   C. 20% of cases
   D. 30% of cases
   E. 50% of cases

THE FOLLOWING STATEMENT CONSISTS OF A STATEMENT AND A REASON. ANSWER BY USING THE FOLLOWING KEY:

   A. If both statement and reason are true and related, cause and effect
   B. If both statement and reason are true, but not related
   C. If the statement is true, but the reason is false
   D. If the statement is false, but the reason is true
   E. If both statement and reason are false

4. It is important to rule out vesicoureteral reflux prior to surgery of ureteropelvic junction obstruction BECAUSE reflux can sometimes be an etiologic factor in obstruction of the ureteropelvic junction.

5. Which of the following operations is best suited for all types of ureteropelvic junction obstruction?
   A. Foley's Y-V plasty
   B. Spiral flap of Culp
   C. Davis intubated ureterotomy
   D. Dismembered pyeloplasty of Anderson-Hynes
   E. Vertical flap of Scardino

ANSWERS AND DISCUSSION

1. (E) All of the answers given here should be included in the differential diagnosis of flank masses in children. They are often difficult to differentiate on physical examination, since all may feel quite firm and irregular. Indeed, the child in this case was referred to us with a diagnosis of Wilms' tumor.

2. (A) If the child is placed in a dark room and a strong light, such as a fiber optic source, is used, a hydronephrotic sac can be transilluminated surprisingly well. It is difficult or impossible to differentiate tumor or cyst on the basis of firmness or irregularity. Hydronephrosis can, at times, be massive and extend across the midline.

3. (C) A recent Mayo Clinic series of 152 children with ureteropelvic junction obstruction revealed bilateral disease in 18% of cases.

4. (A) Hutch pointed out many years ago that what appears to be classical ureteropelvic junction obstruction can, at times, be caused by massive reflux. With the added load of the refluxing urine, the ureteropelvic junction becomes relatively decompensated and unable to pass this increased volume back down to the bladder. Although this is a rare cause, it should always be ruled out. Occasionally, both problems are found to be present simultaneously, and some have advocated repairing both conditions at the same time.[4]

5. (D) The five types of plastic repair commonly used for this procedure are listed here. Each has its indications and advocates. However, most surgeons would agree that the dismembered pyeloplasty of Anderson and Hynes lends itself best to repair of all abnormalities found at the ureteropelvic junction.

REFERENCES, CASES 6 AND 7

1. Culp OS: Choice of operations for ureteropelvic obstruction: A review of 385 cases. Can J Surg 4:157-165, 1961.

2. Zincke H, Kelalis PP, and Culp OS: Ureteropelvic junction obstruction in children. Surg, Gyn and Obstet 139:873, Dec. 1974.

3. Dwoskin J: Management of the massively dilated urinary tract in infants by temporary diversion and single-stage reconstruction. Urol Clin N Amer 1:515, 1974.

4. Stewart BH: Operative Urology, Williams and Wilkins Company, Baltimore, 1975, Chapter 11, p. 152.

CASE 8: 32-YEAR-OLD MALE WITH DIFFICULTY VOIDING

HISTORY

A 32-year-old male was seen because of great difficulty in voiding for the past six months. He stated that, one and one-half years previously, he had fulguration of condyloma acuminata of the urethral meatus, as well as the penile urethra. He had some slowing of the urinary stream since that time, but it had become considerably worse over the past several months. He had to strain severely to void, and had frequency every 2 hours during the day and nocturia several times. He stated his urinary stream was very thin. There was no dysuria or history of urinary tract infection.

PHYSICAL EXAMINATION

There was no evidence of recurrent condyloma acuminata. The entire physical examination was within normal limits. He was observed voiding with a very slow stream.

LABORATORY DATA

Urine analysis revealed 4-8 WBC per high power field; otherwise normal. Urine culture showed no growth after 48 hours. BUN, creatinine normal. Intravenous urogram revealed normal upper tracts. The excretory cystogram was normal, and there was a moderate amount of residual urine. Urine flowmetry revealed an average flow rate of 1.75cc/sec and a maximum flow rate of 2cc/sec. It took him over 3.5 minutes to void 400cc (Fig. 8.1). A retrograde urethrogram showed a short stricture of the distal urethral bulb (Fig. 8.2). Antegrade urethrogram confirmed the same short stricture.

CLINICAL COURSE

The patient absolutely refused urethral dilatations, and so underwent urethroplasty by resection of the short stricture and end-to-end anastomosis of the spatulated urethral ends. His postoperative course was entirely uneventful, and he voided with an excellent stream after removal of the catheter. A postoperative urine flowmetry revealed an average flow of 26cc/sec with a maximum flow of 44cc/sec (see Fig. 8.1B).

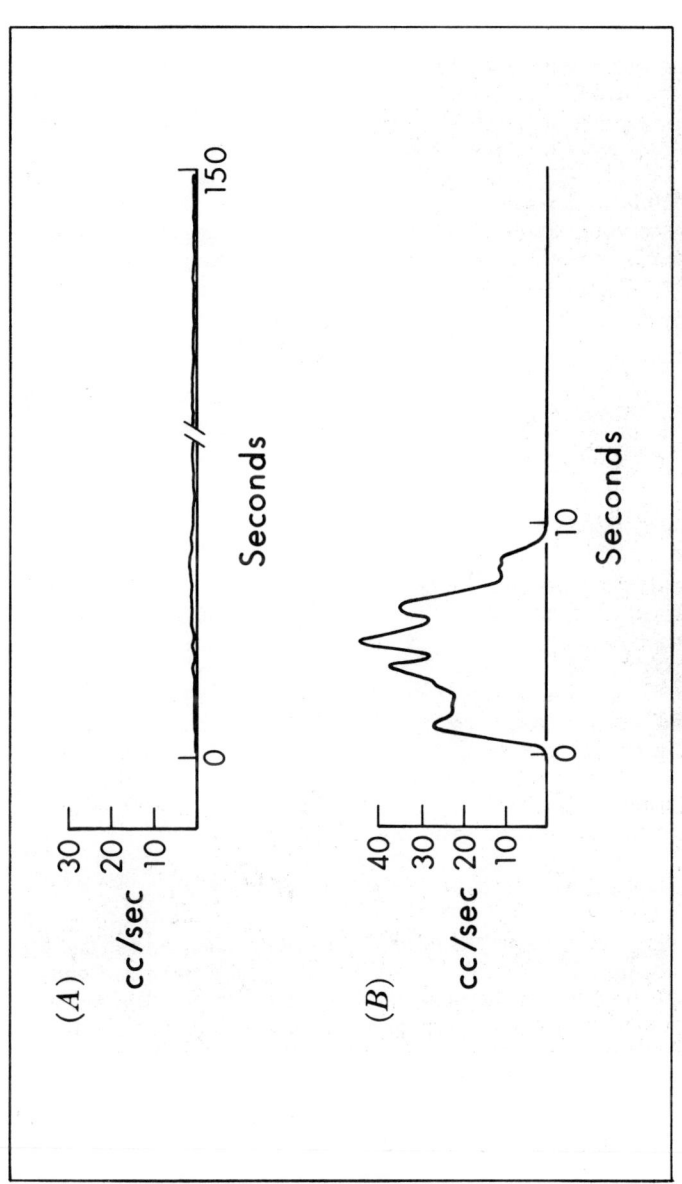

FIG. 8.1: (A) Urine flowmetry pre-op: Average flow - 1.75cc/sec; Maximum flow - 2cc/sec. (B) Urine flowmetry post-op: Average flow - 26cc/sec; Maximum flow - 44cc/sec.

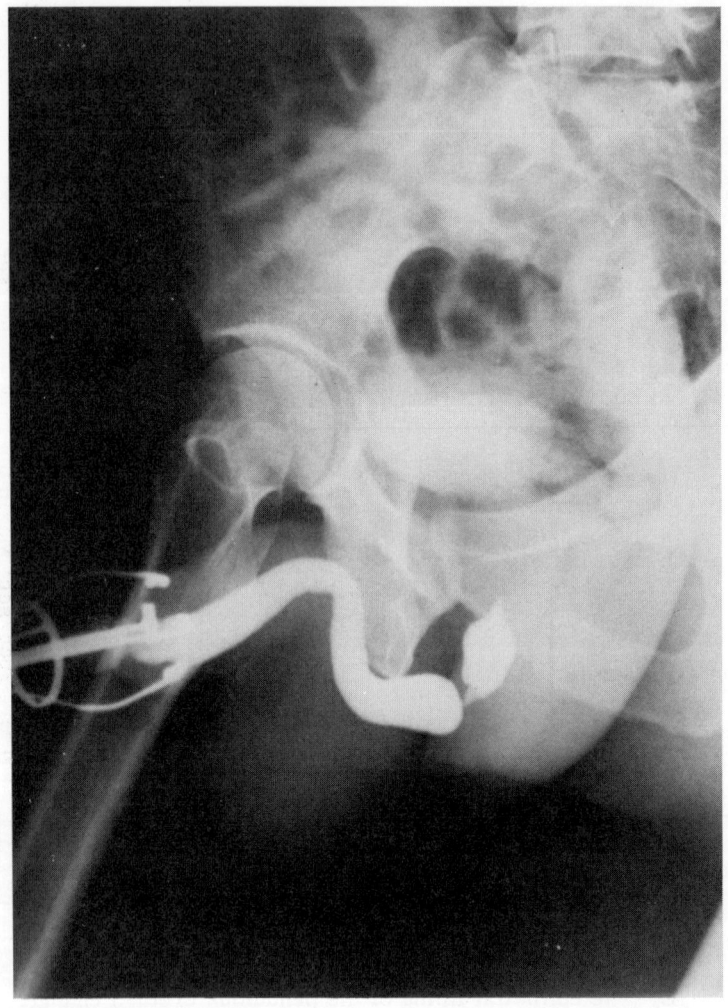

FIG. 8.2: Retrograde urethrogram shows a short stricture of the distal bulbous urethra.

Urinary Obstruction

QUESTIONS

1. The majority of strictures are best treated by:
   A. Johansen urethroplasty
   B. Devine procedure
   C. Urethral dilatations
   D. Turner-Warwick urethroplasty
   E. Blandy urethroplasty

2. The most common cause of urethral stricture today is:
   A. Postgonococcal infection
   B. Posttraumatic secondary to external injury
   C. Postsurgical-iatrogenic

3. The membranous urethra is lined by:
   A. Transitional epithelium
   B. Stratified squamous epithelium
   C. Stratified columnar epithelium
   D. Simple columnar epithelium
   E. B & C

4. The pendulous urethra is lined by:
   A. Transitional epithelium
   B. Stratified squamous epithelium
   C. Stratified columnar epithelium
   D. Simple columnar epithelium
   E. B & C

ANSWERS AND DISCUSSION

1. (C) The great majority of urethral strictures are best managed by regular and gentle dilatation. As time progresses, the intervals between dilatations should become progressively longer. This patient had had several dilatations in the past and absolutely refused this procedure.

2. (C)

3. (C)

4. (E) The epithelial lining of the pendulous urethra changes from stratified columnar proximally to stratified squamous in its distal portion.

REFERENCES

1. Devine PC, et al.: Use of full thickness skin graft in repair of urethral stricture. J Urol 90:67, 1963.

2. Johansen B: Reconstruction of the male urethra in stricture. ACTA Chir Scand: Suppl 176, 1953.

3. Turner-Warwick RT: A technique for posterior urethroplasty. J Urol 83:416, 1960.

CHAPTER II

GENITOURINARY INJURY

INTRODUCTION

Injuries to the genitourinary organs are becoming more and more common in our fast-moving society. Although these are usually associated with injuries to other parts of the body; in generalized trauma they are occasionally isolated. Treatment of shock and hemorrhage are of primary importance. If possible, a careful history of the circumstances surrounding the accident should be taken, as well as the exact mechanism of injury. Important physical findings pointing to urinary tract injury include ecchymosis over the renal areas, as well as pelvic and perineal region or masses secondary to hemorrhage or urinary extravasation. Blood at the urethral meatus is indicative of urethral injury. Rectal examination in these patients is an essential part of the physical examination. Upward placement of the prostate may indicate a so-called "floating prostate," which has been sheared from its attachment to the membranous urethra. Bogginess in this area could be indicative of hematoma or urinary extravasation.

Special urologic investigation should be carried out as indicated, but only after shock and hemorrhage appear to be under control. We generally do an urethrogram prior to passage of a catheter, if there is blood at the urethral meatus. If there is no gross blood, a catheter is passed. Gross blood in the bladder urine indicates serious injury to the urinary tract. One occasionally finds fat bubbles floating on the surface of the bloody urine, indicating the presence of bladder perforation with fat extruding into the bladder. Cystoscopy and retrograde pyelograms are occasionally helpful, especially in the presence of nonvisualization of one kidney. We have found renal angiography most helpful.

Injuries of the kidney can be classified into:

1. Simple contusions with and without rupture of the capsule
2. Laceration:
    a) parenchymal injuries

b) collecting system injuries
   c) combined
3. Renal pulpification
4. Injuries to the vascular pedicle

Types 1 and 2 can, in the majority of cases, be handled conservatively with bed rest and close observation, even in the presence of moderate amounts of uninfected urinary extravasation.

Types 3 and 4 are best managed surgically. Angiography is probably the best way to differentiate the four types of injury prior to surgery, and is indispensable in some cases for proper management. Late complications of renal injury can include atrophy or fibrosis with or without hypertension. Hydronephrosis secondary to urinary extravasation and periureteral fibrosis is a rare, late complication.

Injuries to the ureter by external violence are very rare, but do occasionally occur. Most reported cases of this type of injury are of young boys being struck by automobiles. Surgical injury to the ureter is not uncommon, however, and may result following abdominal or vaginal hysterectomy, abdominoperineal resection, or anterior resection. Management is dependent on the time of discovery of the injury. If early, direct reanastomosis either ureter-to-ureter, or ureter-to-bladder, would be preferable. If more than several days, and less than 3 months have elapsed, preliminary diversion by nephrostomy or ureterostomy, with a later repair of the injured area, is the preferred method of management.

Bladder injuries can be produced by external violence or can be surgically induced. The former are usually associated with pelvic fractures, but not invariably so, and may be induced by so-called "insignificant amounts of trauma." Ruptured bladders with extravasation are classified into intraperitoneal and extraperitoneal types, and are best handled by primary repair, suprapubic cystotomy and drainage. Some urologists will treat extraperitoneal ruptures caused by transurethral surgery with catheter drainage alone, but this is advisable only in limited circumstances. Surgically induced bladder injuries, especially following gynecologic surgery, can result in vesicovaginal fistula. If the fistula is less than 4mm in diameter, fulguration of the entire tract can be successful in a high number of cases. Vesicovaginal fistula following hysterectomy which is greater than 4mm is best managed by partial colpocleisis (Latzko procedure).

Urethral injuries are divided into those affecting the posterior urethra (above the urogenital diaphragm) and those affecting the anterior urethra. These can be partial or complete transections. In complete transections, surgery is mandatory in order to re-establish continuity of the urinary stream. Interlocking sounds have been used for this purpose, but the direct approach with reanastomosis of the severed portion of urethra is probably best when feasible. In some instances, there is extensive diffuse bleeding and bony injury, making direct anastomosis extremely difficult. In complete transection, if a catheter can be passed into the bladder, it is left indwelling as a splint. Simple diversion of urine in these cases, without extensive x-ray investigation at the time of injury, has been advocated by many. Direct secondary repair 3-4 months later can be undertaken, and the long-term complications of stricture and impotence have been reported to be excellent in these cases.

CASE 9: 16-YEAR-OLD MALE WITH INJURY TO LEFT FLANK

HISTORY

This 16-year-old white male was admitted with a chief complaint of gross hematuria following injury in the left flank. The patient injured his left side when he hit a tree while sledding. He also injured his left hand, and sustained a fracture of the metacarpal bones. He denied dysuria, frequency, or other urinary complaints.

PAST MEDICAL HISTORY

He had tonsillectomy at age 12. There was no history of allergy. Review of systems was negative.

PHYSICAL EXAMINATION

On admission, temperature 37.2° centigrade; pulse 80 and regular; respirations 20 per minute; blood pressure 130/80. He was in no distress and was quite cooperative. There was left CVA tenderness and a mass palpable in the left flank. There was no suprapubic tenderness.

LABORATORY DATA

Urine showed gross hematuria. Hematocrit 44%; WBC, electrolytes, normal. BUN 13 mg%; glucose 105 mg%. Hand films revealed fracture of the 2nd, 4th and 5th metacarpals. Chest x-ray was normal.

QUESTIONS

1. The next step in the care of this patient should be:
   A. Complete bed rest
   B. Operate immediately
   C. Intravenous urogram
   D. Cystoscopy to see where gross blood is coming from
   E. Treat with intravenous fluids and operate in 3-4 days

Intravenous urogram revealed prompt bilateral excretion, with what appeared to be a laceration of the left mid-kidney (Figs. 9.1 and 9.2). Retrograde ureteropyelogram was normal, with no evidence of extravasation. Renal angiogram revealed a normal angiographic pattern with an area of radiolucency in the mid-portion of the left kidney, indicating a complete laceration (Fig. 9.3).

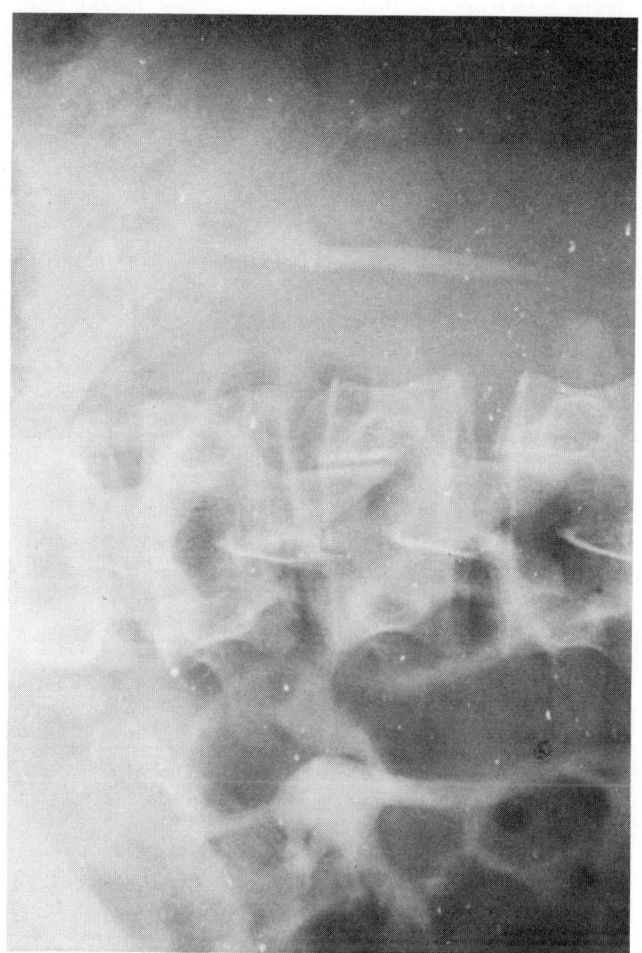

FIG. 9.1: Intravenous urogram. There is a decrease in concentration of contrast material in the mid-portion of the left kidney.

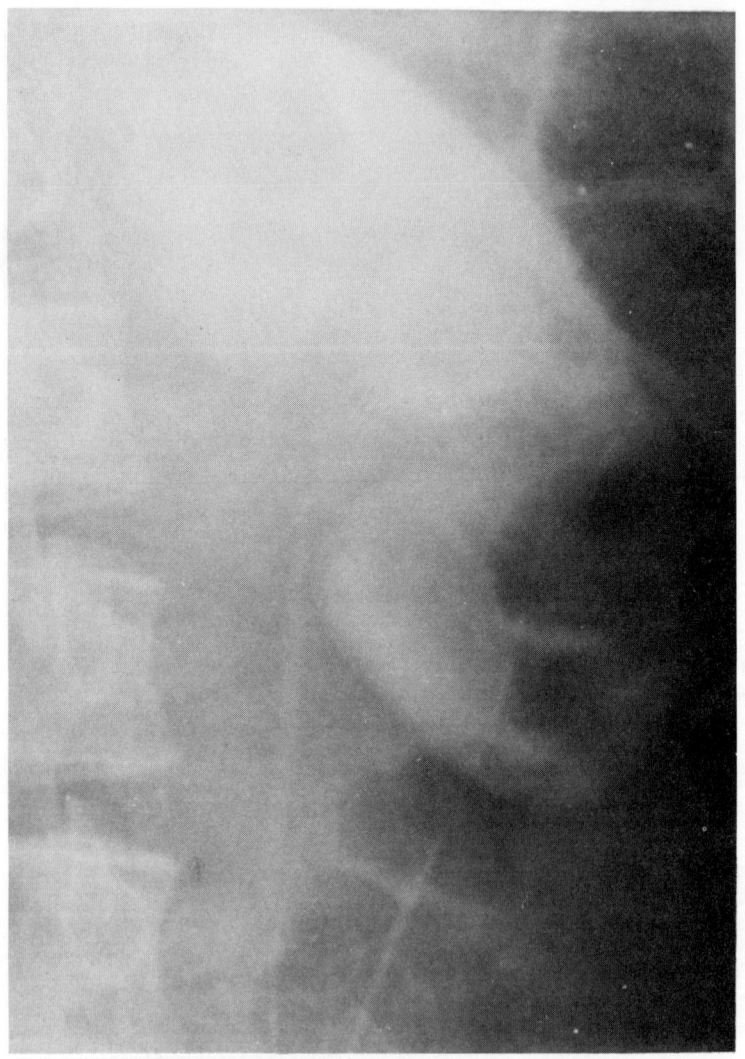

FIG. 9.2: Nephrogram showing decreased concentration in linear area in mid-kidney.

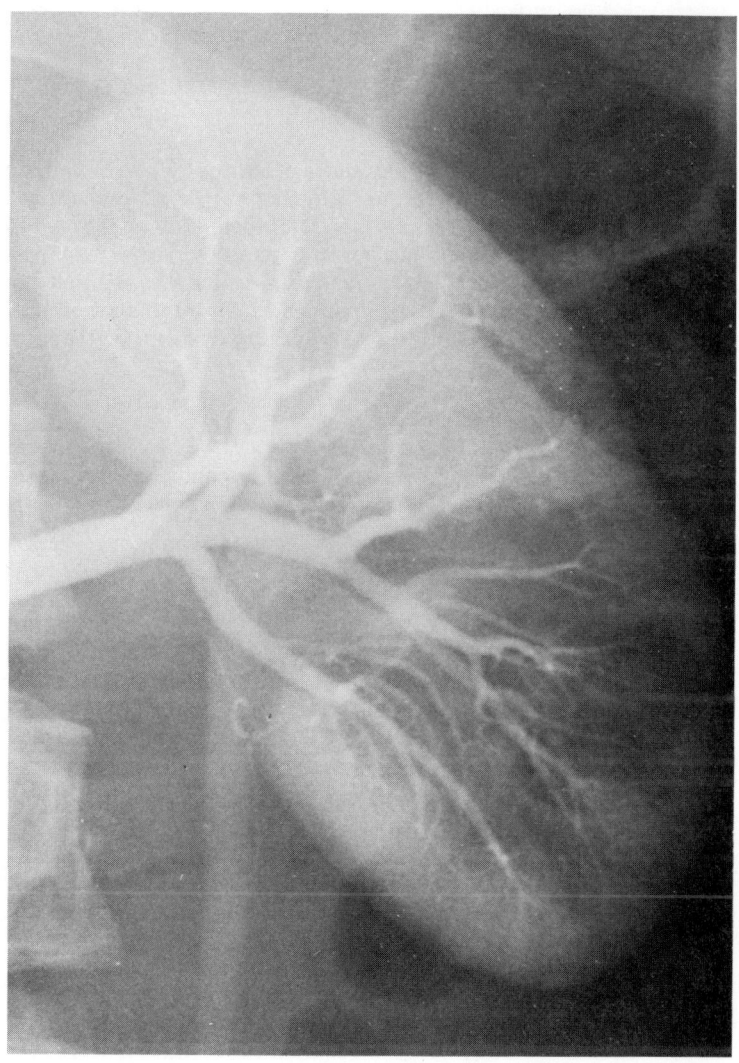

FIG. 9.3: Selective angiogram. There is a normal angiographic pattern with an area of radiolucency in the mid-portion of the left kidney, indicating a laceration at this point.

2. Proper therapy at this point should be:
   A. Complete bed rest
   B. Immediate surgery
   C. Blood transfusion and delayed surgery
   D. Ambulation ad lib with close observation

CLINICAL COURSE

The patient was put on bed rest and antibiotics. The hematocrit dropped from 44% to 38% on the following day, but he required no blood transfusions. Vital signs remained stable. The left CVA tenderness persisted without any mass palpable. He remained at bed rest for 2 weeks, and was ambulated without further bleeding. Intravenous urogram 3 weeks later showed normal functioning and normal right collecting system, without evidence of extravasation.

3. Retroperitoneal hematomas:
   A. Should always be explored
   B. If explored, may convert a benign condition into massive hemorrhage
   C. Do not cause ileus
   D. Generally become infected

EACH OF THE FOLLOWING STATEMENTS CONSISTS OF A STATEMENT AND A REASON. ANSWER BY USING THE FOLLOWING KEY:

   A. If both statement and reason are true and related, cause and effect
   B. Statement and reason are true, but unrelated
   C. Statement true, reason false
   D. Statement false, reason true
   E. Statement and reason are false

4. The conservative management of most renal injuries has become the treatment of choice BECAUSE antibiotic therapy has decreased the incidence of infection.

5. Transverse tears with subcapsular hemorrhage always require immediate surgery BECAUSE these injuries always lead to hypertension.

6. Rupture of the kidney may be associated with clear urine BECAUSE the tear may not involve the collecting system.

Genitourinary Injury   Case 9/ 53

7. The degree of hematuria is an important sign in renal injury BECAUSE the degree of hematuria correlates directly with the degree of injury.

ANSWERS AND DISCUSSION

1. (C) The intravenous urogram is the primary examination in trauma to the upper tract. This not only gives us an idea of the extent of injury on the affected side, but just as important, one sees the condition of the opposite kidney as well. Rarely, a solitary kidney is injured, and this would be most essential to ascertain early. On occasion, the contralateral kidney may be found to be suboptimal in function, or may harbor pre-existing disease. This would certainly change the course of therapy. The initial IVP in trauma should be by high dose infusion technique with tomography.

2. (A) The great majority of renal injuries can be treated conservatively with bed rest, and bleeding will cease spontaneously. Even with severe laceration such as seen here, as long as the patient's condition remains stable and there is no sign of continued blood loss, bed rest with careful observation would be the best treatment. Only 10-20% of cases of renal injury require early surgical intervention.

3. (B) The presence of a retroperitoneal hematoma does not, in and of itself, require evacuation. These often tamponade the bleeding point and the bleeding becomes self-limited. Often, evacuation of the hematoma causes resumption of massive hemorrhage, with control then becoming very difficult and nephectomy being required to control hemorrhage. If possible, vascular control of the renal pedicle should be obtained with noncrushing clamps prior to evacuation of a retroperitoneal hematoma.

4. (B) Both statements are true, but antibiotics or infection are not the sole reason for this. As stated earlier, most renal injuries will stop hemorrhaging with mere bed rest and most will be uncomplicated.

5. (E) Subcapsular hemorrhage generally tamponades itself because of the limited space for an expanding hemorrhage. Although some renal injuries may lead to hypertension as a long-term complication, the incidence after simple subcapsular hematoma must be very low.

6. (A)

7. (E) Oftentimes, microscopic hematuria can be associated with the most severe of renal injuries, and large amounts of blood in the urine may be seen with injuries requiring only conservative management. In general, the degree of hematuria does not correlate well with the degree of injury.

Genitourinary Injury

CASE 10: 17-YEAR-OLD MALE WITH STAB WOUNDS

HISTORY

This 17-year-old male drug addict was admitted on January 10, 1971, after sustaining stab wounds to the right posterolateral chest. These were associated with gross hematuria. In the emergency room, it was felt he had a right hemopneumothorax, and 2 chest tubes were inserted into the right lateral chest.

PAST MEDICAL HISTORY

Skull fracture as a child; gonorrhea twice during the last year prior to admission.

PHYSICAL EXAMINATION

Blood pressure 100/60; pulse 100; respirations 20. The examination of the chest revealed decreased breath sounds bilaterally. There were 2 chest tubes in place on the right side with a stab wound in the right posterolateral 8th intercostal space. The heart was normal. The abdomen was distended with diffuse guarding and rigidity. There was fullness and tenderness in the right upper quadrant, and tenderness in the right lower quadrant. There was right CVA tenderness. There were stab wounds over the 11th rib in the posterior axillary line. The extremities revealed evidence of needle tracks. Renal examination was negative, no masses were palpable.

LABORATORY DATA

Hematocrit 28%; WBC 15,800; urinalysis showed grossly bloody urine. Chest x-ray revealed an elevated right hemidiaphragm. Intravenous urogram showed prompt bilateral excretion with marked extravasation of contrast material on the right side (Fig. 10.1).

QUESTIONS

1. Proper management at this point should be:
    A. Immediate surgery through a flank incision
    B. Blood transfusion and delayed surgery
    C. Bed rest with careful observation
    D. Immediate surgery through an anterior abdominal incision
    E. I.V. fluids and antibiotics

2. At surgery, a huge retroperitoneal hematoma was seen. Proper course of action would be:

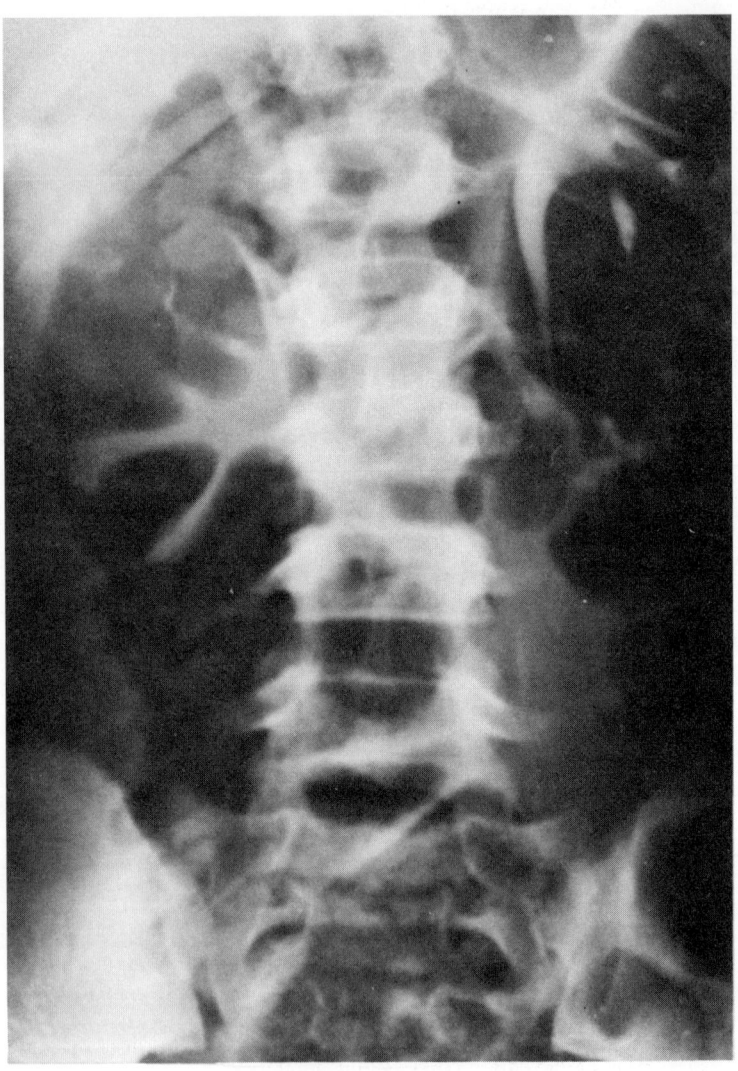

FIG. 10.1: Intravenous urogram showing marked urinary extravasation on the right.

Genitourinary Injury

A. Immediate evacuation of hematoma
B. Placement of vascular clamp on right renal artery and exploration of kidney
C. Immediate right nephrectomy
D. Placement of drain in retroperitoneum with exploration
E. Leave the hematoma alone to avoid further bleeding

CLINICAL COURSE

Patient was immediately explored through a long midline incision over the abdomen. There was a huge right retroperitoneal hematoma of about 1500cc pushing the colon, duodenum, and abdominal viscera anteromedially. The right kidney was torn at the point between the upper 2/3 and the lower 1/3 almost through its complete thickness. There were also lacerations of the right hemidiaphragm and liver. Because of profuse bleeding from the kidney, a right nephrectomy was performed, and the liver and diaphragmatic lacerations were sutured. Postoperative course was benign, and the chest tubes were removed on the 3rd postoperative day. The nasogastric tube was removed on the 4th postoperative day, and the patient made an uneventful recovery.

EACH OF THE FOLLOWING STATEMENTS CONSISTS OF A STATEMENT AND A REASON. ANSWER BY USING THE FOLLOWING KEY:

A. If statement and reason are true and related
B. If statement and reason are true and unrelated
C. If statement true, reason false
D. If statement false, reason true
E. If both statement and reason are false

3. All patients with penetrating injury to the kidney should be subjected to exploratory laparotomy BECAUSE most of them will have an associated intra-abdominal injury.

4. Penetrating renal injuries are best treated conservatively without surgery BECAUSE the injury is usually mild.

5. The incidence of secondary hemorrhage is higher in penetrating renal injury than in nonpenetrating BECAUSE the bleeding is not tamponaded as well in the latter type.

6. Infection is higher in penetrating injury BECAUSE these are almost always contaminated.

ANSWERS AND DISCUSSION

1. (D) This patient had penetrating stab wounds to the abdomen. Although these were posterior, he also had guarding and rigidity of the abdomen, making exploratory laparotomy mandatory. Therefore, a midline incision would be the one of choice. Indeed, the patient did have a liver laceration which was repaired.

2. (B) The best course of action would have been placement of a vascular clamp on the right renal artery. This can be accomplished by rotation of the second portion of the duodenum medially, thus exposing the right renal vessels. After clamping the artery, the hematoma can then be evacuated and bleeding point noted. Suture ligatures can be placed and, if possible, only removal of a portion of the kidney can be done. In this case, it may have been helpful to have a renal angiogram preoperatively. However, the poor condition of the patient precluded this. At times, in the presence of massive retroperitoneal hemorrhage, exposure of the renal artery may be very difficult.

    Had the bleeding been less in Case 10, partial nephrectomy might have been attempted, but time was of the essence here and, although nephrectomy was radical treatment, it was life saving, and the only thing that could have been done under the circumstances.

3. (A) At least 80% of patients with penetrating renal injuries have associated intra-abdominal injuries and, therefore, we believe all patients with penetrating injuries should have surgical exploration.

4. (E) Penetrating injuries are best treated by early surgery because:

    a) there is usually an associated intra-abdominal injury;
    b) tamponading is not always present because of penetration of Gerota's fascia;
    c) they are often contaminated.

5. (A) As stated above, if Gerota's fascia is penetrated, allowing a continuous leak from this space, tamponade of the bleeding site cannot occur.

6. (A)

CASE 11: 11-YEAR-OLD BOY HIT BY AUTOMOBILE

HISTORY

This patient is an 11-year-old boy who was admitted to the hospital after being struck by an automobile.

PHYSICAL EXAMINATION

Blood pressure 128/70; pulse 124 per minute, and temperature 101°. There was diffuse tenderness over the right side of the pubis. The abdomen was soft, with no guarding or rebound tenderness. There was a laceration of the left forehead. The remainder of the physical examination was unremarkable.

LABORATORY DATA

The urine was grossly clear, but many red blood cells were found in the sediment. The hemogram was normal. BUN 16 mg%. An excretory urogram showed prompt excretion bilaterally, with marked extravasation of contrast material from the left ureter (Fig. 11.1). Both calyceal systems appeared normal.

QUESTIONS

1. A diagnostic procedure that may be helpful in this case would be:
   A. Cystogram and voiding cystourethrogram
   B. Cystoscopy and retrograde ureterogram
   C. Aortography and renal angiogram
   D. Renal scan
   E. Sonography

2. Urinary extravasation in blunt renal trauma requires:
   A. Immediate surgery and drainage
   B. Immediate repair of renal injury
   C. Is not, in and of itself, an indication for surgery
   D. Nephrectomy
   E. Passage of a ureteral catheter

CLINICAL COURSE

The left kidney was immediately explored through a classical flank incision. There was a large collection of urine in the retroperitoneal space. The kidney appeared normal. The ureter was completely severed approximately 1cm distal to the ureteropelvic junction. The severed ends were approximated by end-to-

Case 11 — Genitourinary Injury

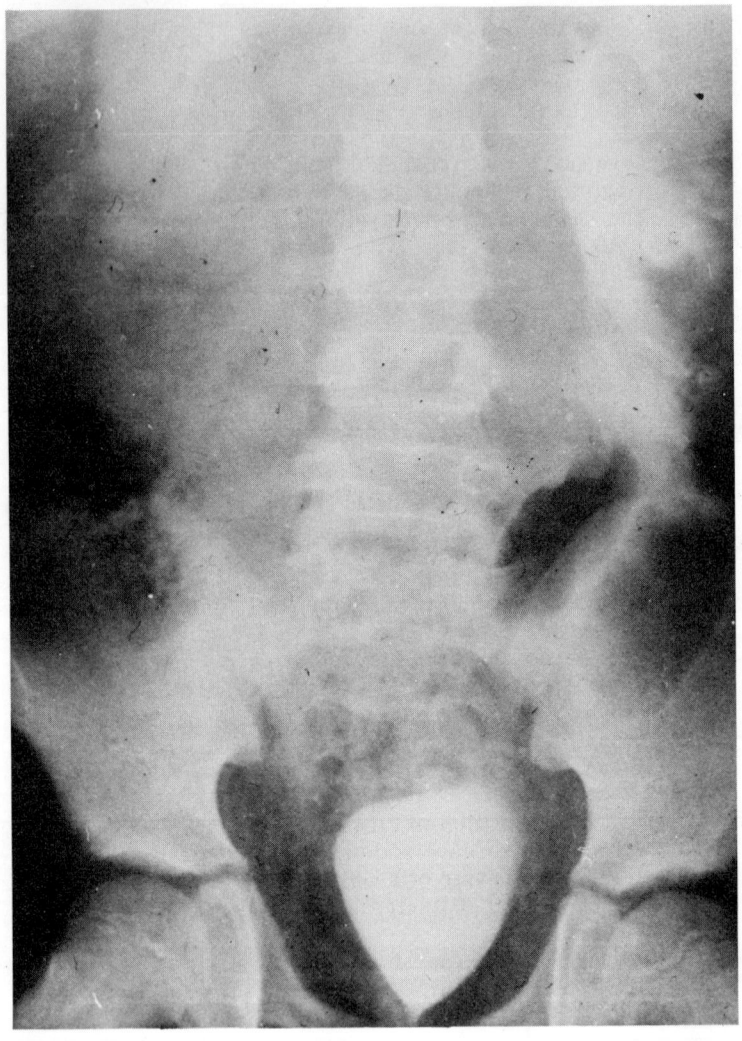

FIG. 11.1: Intravenous urogram. There is extravasation of contrast material from upper left ureter (right side of picture).

Genitourinary Injury

Case 11/ 61

end ureteroureterostomy using #5-0 chromic catgut over a polyethylene splint. The area was drained with a Penrose drain. Postoperative course was uneventful, and the child has done well to this date. An intravenous urogram 3 months postoperatively was normal with no evidence of obstruction; it is shown in Fig. 11.2.

3. Which of the following may be important in healing of the ureter?
   A. Inadequate debridement of injury
   B. Urinary leakage through anastomosis
   C. Use of excessive suture material
   D. Tension on the anastomosis
   E. All of the above

4. Injury to middle third of the ureter can be treated easiest by:
   A. End-to-end anastomosis
   B. Ureteroneocystostomy
   C. Ureteropyelostomy
   D. Autotransplantation
   E. Ureteral substitution with ileum

ANSWERS AND DISCUSSION

1. (B) Although not performed in this case, a retrograde ureterogram would have given a definitive preoperative diagnosis, in this case showing the complete disruption of the ureter. In the year this child was seen, it was generally felt that urinary extravasation meant mandatory drainage and, since the child was to be explored anyway, this procedure was not done. It can be seen on the urogram that the collecting system appears to be normal, so that angiography would probably not have been helpful here. Renal scan has been of limited usefulness in our hands in the acute management of renal injury. However, they are very useful in following patients on a day-to-day basis.

2. (C) In the absence of severe hemorrhage or infection necessitating surgery, a small-to-moderate amount of minor extravasation is not, in and of itself, an indication for surgery. Extravasation from the pelvis or infundibulum, as long as it is not progressive, can heal quite well. The patient must be watched carefully, however, for signs of infection, urinoma, and decreasing renal function. In this situation, periodic renal scans may be quite helpful.

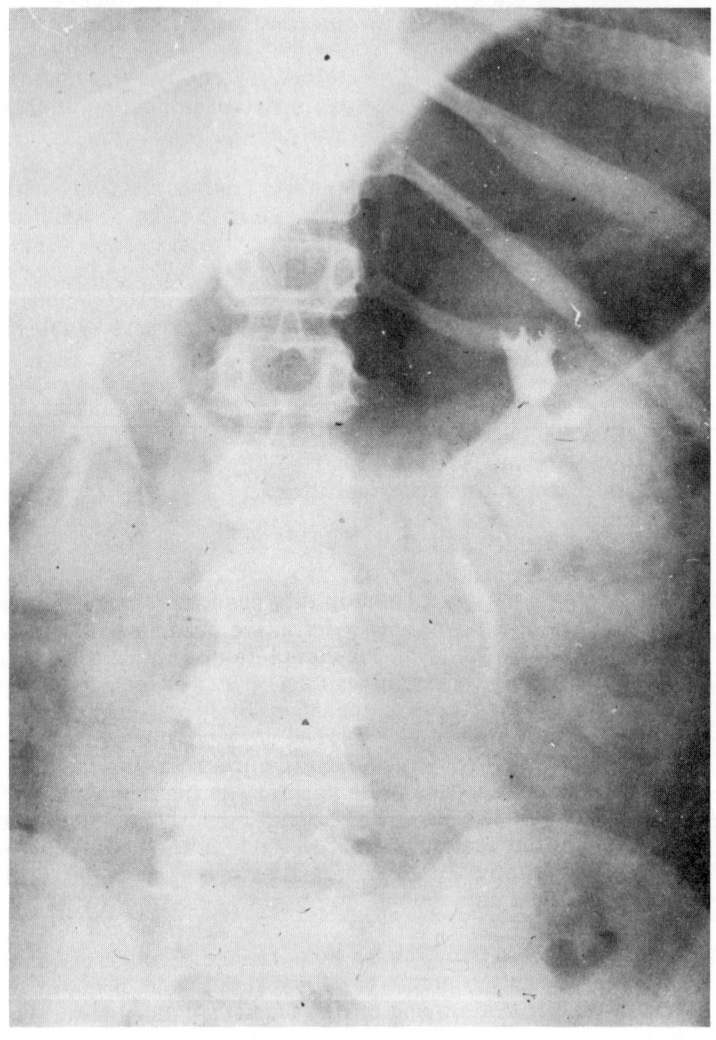

FIG. 11.2: Intravenous urogram, 3 months postoperatively.

3. (E) Development of a ureteral stricture after repair of a ureteral injury can be secondary to any, or a combination of all, factors mentioned. Injured ends of the ureters must be adequately debrided to avoid sloughing of devitalized ends. Urinary leakage through the anastomosis may give rise to periureteritis and scar formation. Excessive suture material will compromise the blood supply, and lead to scar or disruption. Tension on the suture line, as in any other suture line, may lead to disruption.

4. (A) Injuries to the middle third of the ureter are best handled by end-to-end anastomosis. The kidney could be mobilized for ureteropyelostomy, but this would risk undue tension on the suture line. A bladder flap would have to be raised (if this is possible) for ureteroneocystostomy. Autotransplantation is possible, but certainly not the simplest solution.

In performing end-to-end anastomosis, the ends must first be debrided very carefully. They are then spatulated, so as to widen the lumen, and closed with 5-0 chromic catgut by either running or interrupted sutures. The anastomosis should then be placed so that abundant retroperitoneal fat completely surrounds it. The use of stents and diversion by nephrostomy is highly controversial at this time, and beyond the scope of this review. Diversion above the anastomosis can be accomplished by a simple slash in the ureter with placement of an adjacent drain.

REFERENCES

1. Fruchtman B and Newman H: Upper ureteral avulsion secondary to nonpenetrating injury. J Urol 93:452, 1965.

2. Carlton CE, Scott R, and Guthrie AG: The initial management of ureteral injuries: A report of 78 cases. J Urol 105:335, 1971.

CASE 12: 41-YEAR-OLD FEMALE WITH FEVER AND URINARY LEAKAGE, POSTHYSTERECTOMY

HISTORY

A 41-year-old female was admitted to the hospital because of abnormal Pap smear on a routine physical examination. She was totally asymptomatic. Past history included right cervical node biopsy in 1968, with diagnosis of tuberculosis, for which she received triple therapy. She had a tubal ligation in 1967, and an appendectomy in 1968.

PHYSICAL EXAMINATION

Entirely negative.

LABORATORY DATA

Urinalysis, culture, blood urea nitrogen, FBS and intravenous urogram were all within normal limits.

CLINICAL COURSE

A D&C and cone biopsy of the cervix were performed. Pathologic report was carcinoma in situ and, following this, a modified radical hysterectomy was performed. Bleeding was profuse, necessitating hypogastric artery ligation and left pararectal packing. She received ten units of blood on the table. Postoperatively, she ran a febrile course and, after removal of the vaginal packing, fluid was noted leaking from her vagina.

QUESTIONS

1. At this time, one could make a definitive diagnosis of:
    A. Vesicovaginal fistula
    B. Right ureterovaginal fistula
    C. Left ureterovaginal fistula
    D. All of the above
    E. None of the above

2. If an intravenous urogram at this time showed a normal right kidney and a markedly hydronephrotic left kidney, one could make a definitive diagnosis of:
    A. Left ureterovaginal fistula
    B. Right ureterovaginal fistula
    C. Vesicovaginal fistula
    D. All of the above
    E. None of the above

Genitourinary Injury   Case 12/ 65

Intravenous urogram showed extravasation of contrast material in the region of the pelvic brim on the left side (Fig. 12.1). Instillation of indigo carmine solution into the bladder failed to show blue on a vaginal tampon, indicating there was no leakage from the bladder. The patient was cystoscoped, and a ureteral catheter was passed into the left renal pelvis past the area of fistula. This drained well for the next few days, but she continued to run a fever of 103 to 104 degrees despite vigorous antibiotic therapy. The catheter became plugged on several occasions, and she continued to drain urine per vagina.

A left nephrostomy was performed, using a #20F Malecot catheter. The ureteral catheter was left in as a splint for ten days in the hope that the fistula would close. Postoperatively, she developed a phlebitis and had several pulmonary emboli requiring Heparin therapy. She was finally discharged on left nephrostomy drainage, and remained dry vaginally.

In December 1970, she was readmitted for evaluation and a left ureteropyelogram demonstrated only the lower ureter and the fistula. A left nephrostogram (Fig. 12.2) showed a slightly dilated collecting system, including the ureter down to the sacrum. No contrast material entered the bladder, indicating complete obstruction at this point. A ureteroneocystostomy was performed. The bladder was freed and attached to the left psoas muscle and the ureter implanted into the bladder through a submucosal tunnel. Postoperative course was uneventful. The nephrostomy tube fell out on the 8th postoperative day, with no drainage from the site following this. She was discharged after having Carbenicillin therapy for a Pseudomonas urinary tract infection. Her urine cultures have remained sterile, and she is asymptomatic. An intravenous urogram showed fairly good excretion on the left, with no dilation. The ureter can be seen down to its junction with the bladder (Fig. 12.3). Retrograde cystogram revealed no reflux.

3. Proper therapy for a severed ureter discovered during hysterectomy would be:
   A. Ligation of ureter
   B. Ureteroureterostomy
   C. Transureteroureterostomy
   D. Ureteroneocystostomy
   E. Nephrectomy

4. A 35-year-old female develops a fever of 103° on the tenth day posthysterectomy. Intravenous urogram reveals grade IV hydronephrosis on the right side. Proper therapy would be:

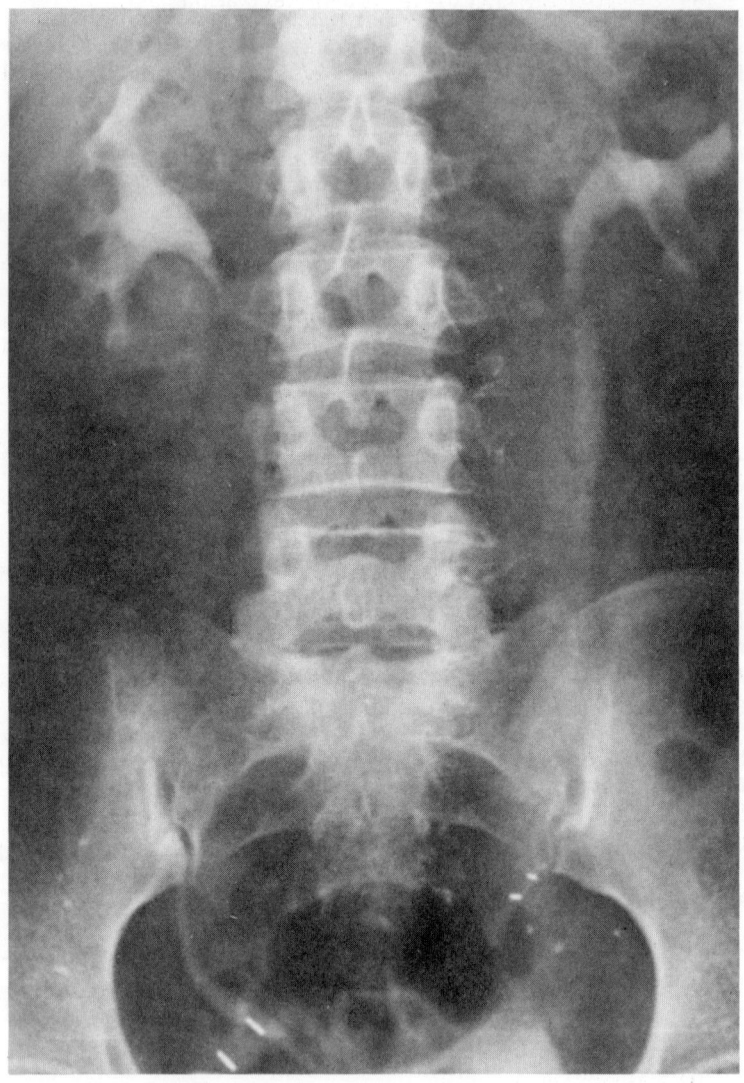

FIG. 12.1: Intravenous urogram following radical hysterectomy. There is extravasation of contrast material in the region of the pelvic brim on the left.

Genitourinary Injury   Case 12/ 67

   A. Immediate right nephrostomy
   B. Immediate right nephrectomy
   C. Cystoscopy and ureteral catheterization
   D. Immediate exploration and ureteroureterostomy
   E. None of the above

5. The above patient is cystoscoped and a catheter cannot be passed beyond 3 cm above the right ureteral orifice. Proper therapy would be:
   A. Immediate right nephrostomy
   B. Immediate right nephrectomy
   C. Exploration and ureteroureterostomy
   D. Transureteroureterostomy
   E. None of the above

6. Ureterovaginal fistula is best diagnosed by:
   A. Intravenous indigo carmine
   B. Intravesical indigo carmine
   C. Intravenous urogram
   D. B plus A
   E. All of the above

ANSWERS AND DISCUSSION

1. (E) All one can say at this point is that there is leakage from the vagina. This may represent urine, or it may be just serous exudate. One could analyze the fluid for urea content to confirm the presence of urine, or one could inject indigo carmine intravenously and, if this appears in the vaginal fluid, then a diagnosis of a urinary fistula can be made. The exact point of fistulization would have to be confirmed by other studies, as outlined in this case.

2. (E) The I.V. urogram, as described in the question, would not indicate where the fistula was coming from. Often, a fistula actually drains an obstructed ureter and what was hydronephrotic prior to the fistula decreases in its degree of obstruction. Therefore, in the hypothetical situation given here, the patient may have a tie on the left ureter, and the fistula may be coming from the apparently normal-looking right ureter. Further studies, i.e., retrograde ureteropyelogram, I.V. indigo carmine, intravesical indigo carmine, etc., would be necessary to make a definitive diagnosis.

3. (D) A ureter which has been severed, and is recognized at the time of surgery, is best managed by reimplantation into the bladder, since this method is associated with fewer

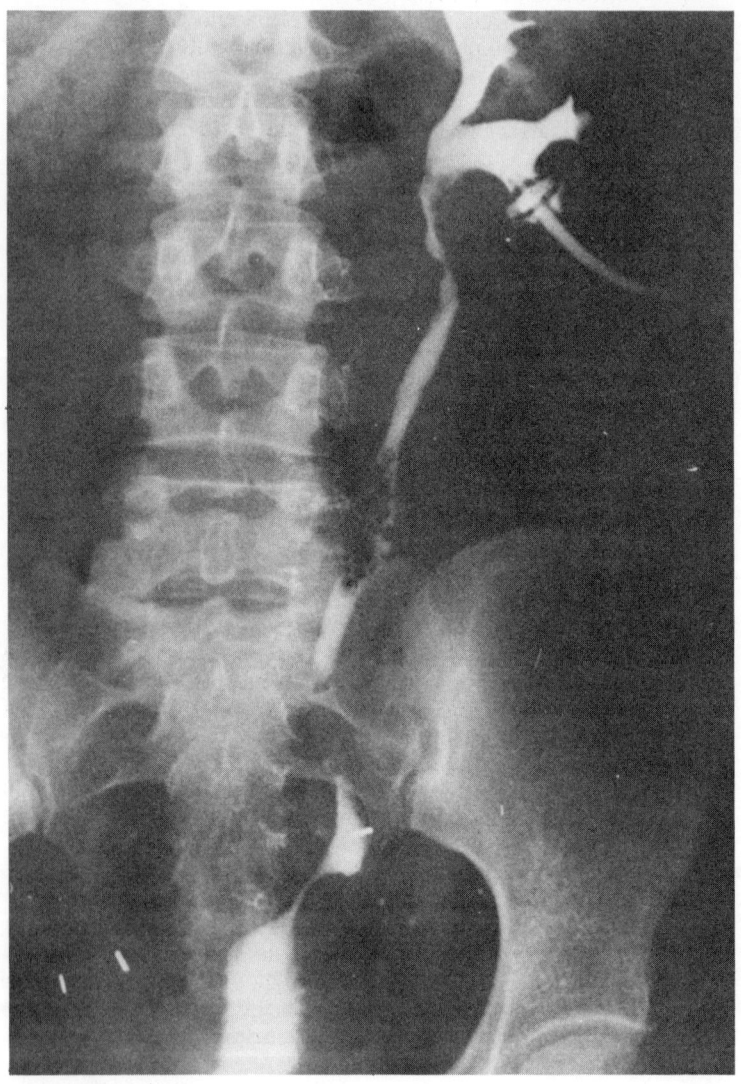

FIG. 12.2: Left nephrostogram. No contrast material enters the bladder, but the vagina is visualized.

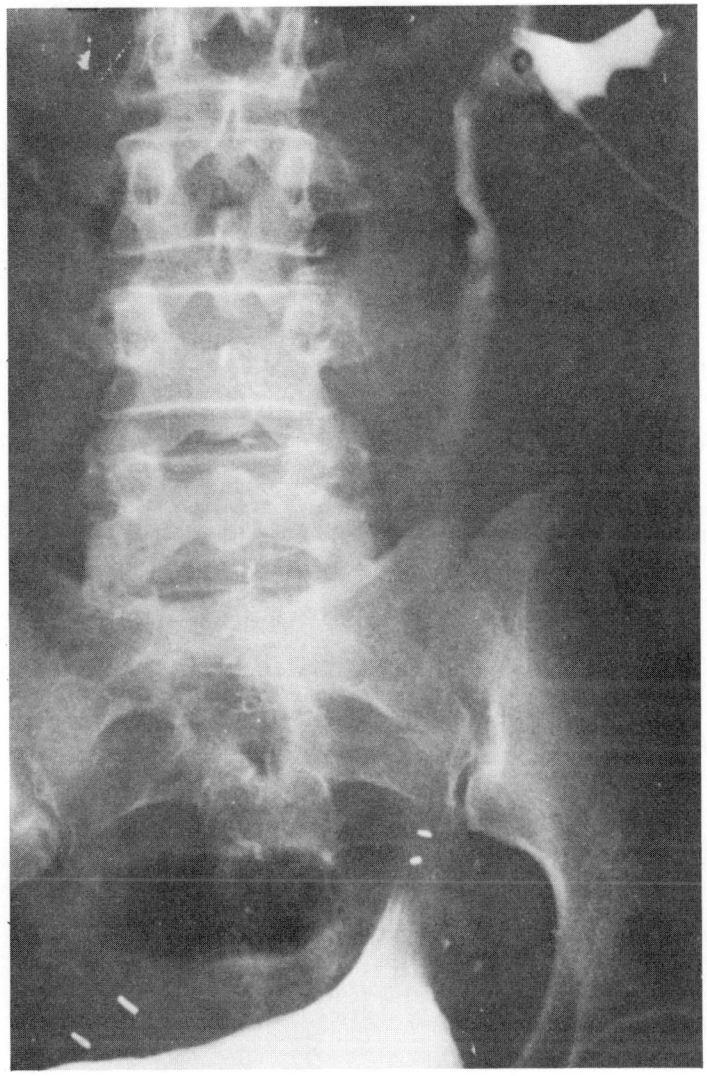

FIG. 12.3: Intravenous urogram, three months after ureteroneocystostomy.

complications than ureteroureterostomy or transureteroureterostomy. The latter have a higher incidence of stricture resulting in obstruction. Although they would be acceptable methods of management, most urologists would agree that reimplantation into the bladder would be preferable, if possible.

4. (C) Initially, attempt at passage of ureteral catheter should be the first thing one should do. If this is successful, it should be left in place for one week and, perhaps, a larger catheter passed for dilatation of the strictured area and drainage of the obstructed kidney. If ureteral catheterization is unsuccessful, and the patient is febrile, some form of urinary drainage and diversion would be mandatory.

5. (A) In a patient who is febrile and ill, and who is more than 4-7 days postoperative, most would agree that urinary diversion by nephrostomy would be the procedure of choice. Some have advocated early direct attack at the obstructed ureter with good result, but they remain in the minority.

6. (D) In the patient with isolated ureterovaginal fistula, the bladder integrity is not lost. If one places a dry tampon in the vagina, and then instills indigo carmine into the bladder, no blue will be noted on the tampon. The bladder is then drained of the dye, and a dose of indigo carmine is then given intravenously. Dye on the tampon at this time, confirms the presence of a ureterovaginal fistula. The site would have to be determined by retrograde ureteropyelograms.

REFERENCES

1. Hach WH, Kursh ED, and Persky L: Early aggressive management of intraoperative ureteral injuries. J Urol 114: 530, Oct. 1975.

2. Weinberg SR, Harmon FL, and Berman R: The management and repair of lesions of the ureter and fistula. Surg Gyn 110:575-584, 1960.

3. Orkin LA: Trauma to the Ureter: Pathogenesis and Management, F.A. Davis, Philadelphia, 1964.

CASE 13: 20-YEAR-OLD MALE WITH ABDOMINAL TRAUMA

HISTORY

This patient is a 20-year-old male, who was struck in the abdomen by his opponents while in a fist fight. He came to the emergency room several hours later complaining of abdominal pain and hematuria.

PHYSICAL EXAMINATION

There was diffuse tenderness and guarding in the entire abdomen. Blood pressure and pulse were normal.

LABORATORY DATA

The urine was grossly bloody. An intravenous urogram was performed which revealed normal upper tracts. Retrograde cystogram showed intraperitoneal extravasation (Fig. 13.1).

CLINICAL COURSE

Exploratory laparotomy was performed. There was no other intraabdominal injury. A 4cm laceration was found in the dome of the bladder and closed with 2 layers from the peritoneal surface. Cystostomy tube was left in place for 14 days. Patient did well postoperatively and has been asymptomatic since discharge.

(T)RUE OR (F)ALSE:

1. Rupture of the bladder caused by a direct blow presupposes a bladder distended with urine.

2. Injuries to the bladder by a direct blow generally result in intraperitoneal tears.

3. Vesical lacerations secondary to fracture of the pelvis generally cause extraperitoneal extravasation.

4. Rupture and perforation of the bladder are fatal injuries unless treated promptly.

ANSWERS AND DISCUSSION

1. (T) A sudden blow to the full bladder causes a very sudden rise in intravesical pressure, which is transmitted equally to all parts of the bladder wall by its fluid contents.

72/ Case 13

Genitourinary Injury

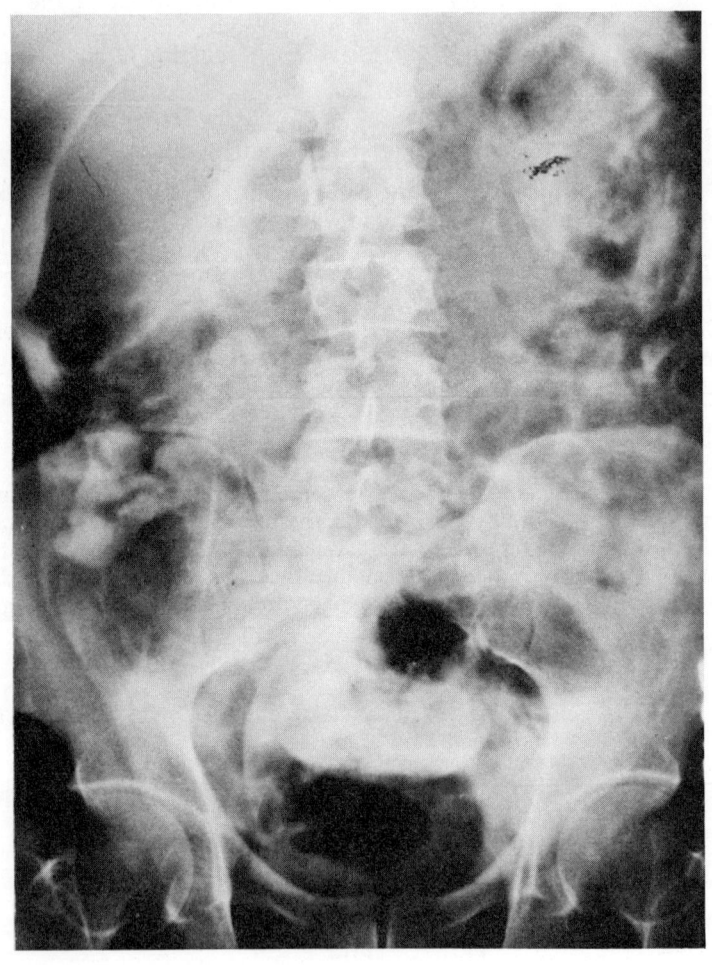

FIG. 13.1: Retrograde cystogram. There is diffuse intraperitoneal extravasation of contrast material.

This may cause either contusion of the wall or complete separation of the wall with perforation.

2. (T) If the force is great enough to cause complete disruption of the bladder wall, this generally occurs at its weakest and least supported part - that is, the dome which is covered by the peritoneal reflection. Rupture through this area results in intraperitoneal extravasation, as illustrated in Fig. 13.1.

3. (T) With fracture of the pubis, it is common for fragments to break off the posterior surface and actually tear through the bladder wall. Since this area of the bladder is below the peritoneal reflection, this will result in an extraperitoneal extravasation.

4. (T) With intraperitoneal perforation, infection of the urine will result in peritonitis and, generally, sepsis and death. In extraperitoneal perforation, a pelvic cellulitis follows an infected urine with abscess formation, sepsis and death, unless adequate drainage is performed.

REFERENCES

1. Reid RE and Herman JR: Rupture of the bladder, urethra: Diagnosis and treatment. NY Med J 65:2685-2696, 1965.

2. Lynch KMJ: Traumatic urinary injuries: Pitfalls in their diagnosis and treatment. J Urol 77:90-95, 1957.

CASE 14: 24-YEAR-OLD MALE WITH GUNSHOT WOUND

HISTORY

A 24-year-old male was brought into the emergency room after being shot three times in a barroom brawl. He had never lost consciousness, but complained of abdominal pain. He had not voided since the incident.

PHYSICAL EXAMINATION

BP 120/74, pulse 100, regular, respirations 20. Chest was clear to percussion and auscultation. The abdomen was soft and nontender and not distended. Bowel sounds were hypoactive. There were three bullet entrance wounds in the left lower quadrant in the inguinal region. No exit wounds could be identified. A voided urine specimen was grossly bloody. Rectal examination was negative.

LABORATORY DATA

Urinalysis was grossly bloody. Hemoglobin and hematocrit were normal.

A plain film of the abdomen showed three bullets in the abdomen, the upper apparently lodged in the muscle of the back on lateral view (Fig. 14.1A). Intravenous urogram revealed normal upper tracts, and the lower bullet appeared to be lodged in the bladder both on AP and oblique views (Fig. 14.1B). A retrograde cystogram revealed extraperitoneal extravasation at the level of the bladder neck (Fig. 14.2).

CLINICAL COURSE

The patient was taken to the operating room immediately, and explored through a midline incision. Intraperitoneal exploration was entirely negative, there being no evidence of injury to the bowel or other intraperitoneal organs.

The bladder was opened, and a 22-caliber bullet was removed from its cavity. A laceration on the left side of the bladder was debrided and repaired and a suprapubic cystostomy tube placed within the bladder. The perivesical space was drained with a Penrose. The patient made an uneventful recovery, and was discharged 15 days postoperatively.

Genitourinary Injury

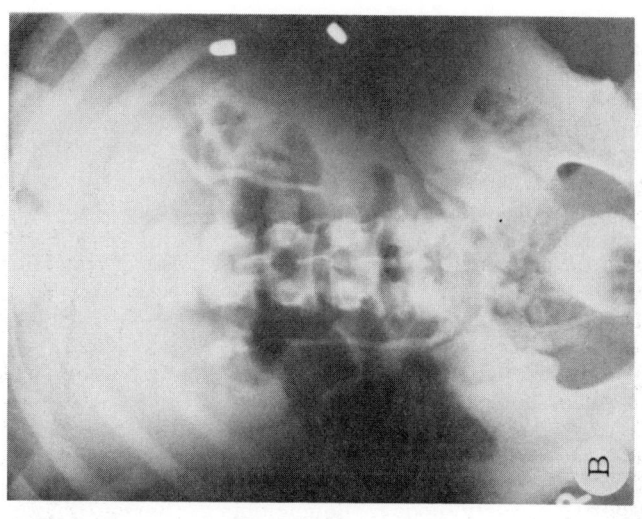
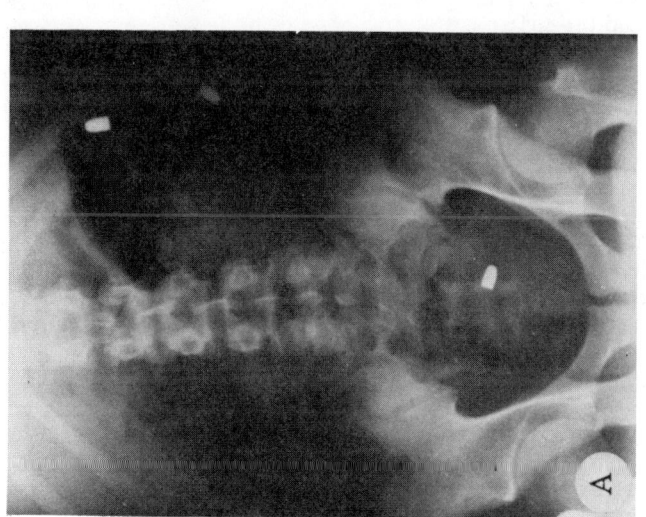

FIG. 14.: (A) Plain film of the abdomen showing two bullets in the left upper quadrant and one in the region of the bladder. (B) Normal intravenous urogram. Lower bullet is within the bladder.

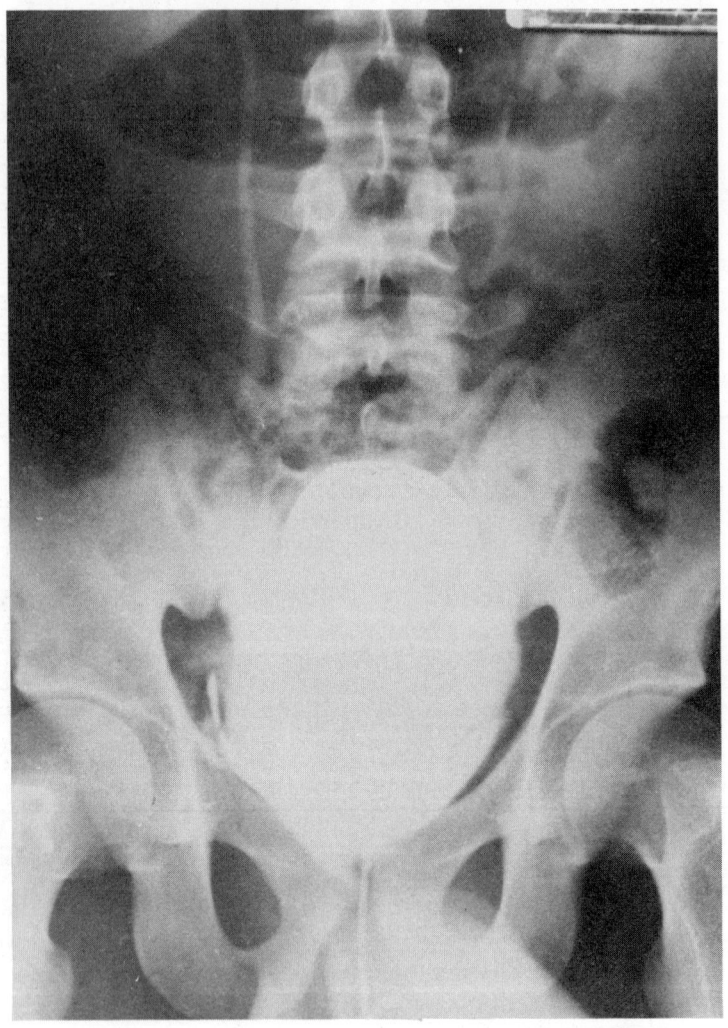

FIG. 14.2: Retrograde cystogram with extraperitoneal extravasation.

Genitourinary Injury   Case 14/ 77

QUESTIONS

1. In a gunshot wound of the abdomen involving both bladder
    and rectosigmoid, proper therapy should include:
    A. Colostomy
    B. Suprapubic cystostomy
    C. Interposition of omentum between bladder and bowel
    D. Drainage of the perivesical space
    E. All of the above

2. If a penetrating injury were near the left ureteral orifice,
    proper therapy should include:
    A. Reimplantation of the left ureter into the bladder
    B. Ureteroureterostomy of the left ureter to the right
    C. Passage of a ureteral catheter
    D. None of the above

ANSWERS AND DISCUSSION

1. (E) In gunshot wounds of the bladder involving the rectum
    or rectosigmoid, both the bladder and colon must be closed
    and a colostomy and a cystostomy performed. If possible,
    some tissue should be interposed between the two injuries
    to prevent fistula formation. Omentum is ideal for this pur-
    pose. Adequate drainage of the perivesical space is impor-
    tant as well.

2. (C) Although major repair may be necessary in this type of
    injury, exploration of the ureter should be carried out first,
    to be sure that correction really is necessary. The passage
    of a ureteral catheter to the renal pelvis will show that ure-
    teral continuity is intact. If there is a question of injury,
    the catheter can be left in place as a stent.

CASE 15: 24-YEAR-OLD MALE WITH PERINEAL INJURY

HISTORY

A 24-year-old male was admitted to the emergency room after sustaining injury to his perineum while working on a ladder. He fell several rungs on the ladder and straddled a lower rung as he fell.

PHYSICAL EXAMINATION

There was blood extruding from the urethral orifice and a hematoma of the perineum. He could not void. There were no other injuries.

QUESTIONS

1. Initial management in this patient would be:
   A. Immediate passage of a Foley catheter
   B. Immediate cystostomy
   C. Insertion of suprapuric catheter with trocar
   D. Retrograde urethrogram
   E. None of the above

2. Retrograde urethrogram in a man with "straddle injury" shows extravasation of contrast material at the bulbous urethra. Proper management would be:
   A. Perineal exploration with attempt at primary closure
   B. Immediate cystostomy
   C. Passage of urethral Foley catheter
   D. Incision and drainage only
   E. None of the above

LABORATORY DATA

An intravenous urogram showed normal upper tracts. Retrograde urethrogram revealed extravasation from the bulbous urethra which was limited by Buck's fascia (Fig. 15.1). The urethral catheter could not be passed in the emergency room.

CLINICAL COURSE

After adequate preparation, he was taken to the operating room, anesthetized and prepared for perineal exploration of the area and possible excision of the injured urethra and end-to-end anastomosis. A #18 French catheter was passed easily into the bladder after preparation. It was left indwelling for 10 days

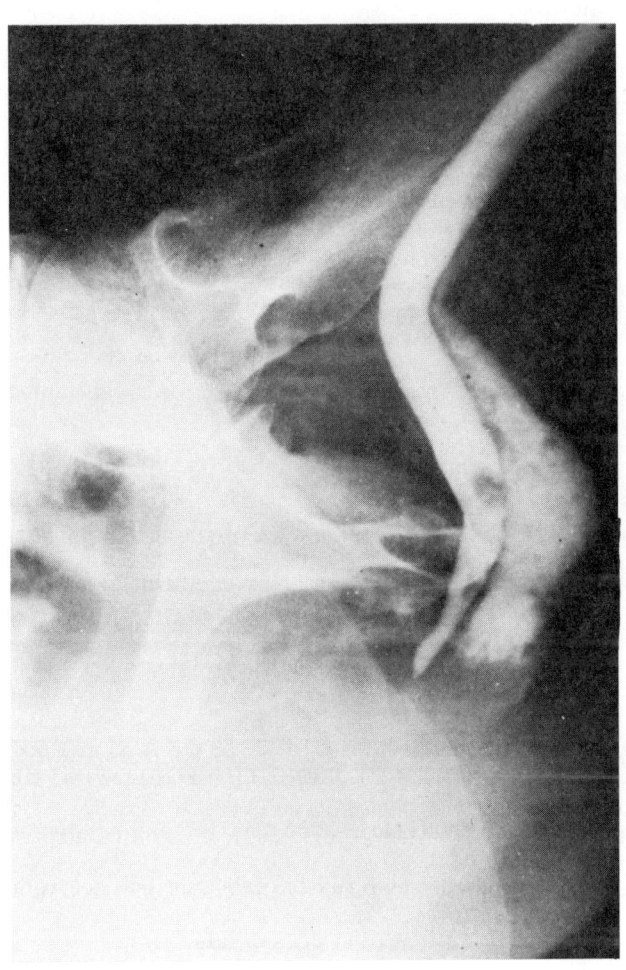

FIG. 15.1: Retrograde urethrogram showing extravasation from the bulbous urethra limited by Buck's fascia.

and gradually increased to #22 French. The catheter was removed and he voided well and made an uneventful recovery. The urethra calibrated easily to #22 French, three months later, and a voiding cystourethrogram was normal.

3. A urethral injury which penetrates Buck's fascia would show the following:
   A. Extravasation into the scrotum
   B. Extravasation into the perineum
   C. Edema of the penis
   D. Extravasation onto the abdominal wall
   E. All of the above

4. The cardinal sign of anterior urethral injury is:
   A. Hematoma of the penis
   B. Tenderness in the perineum
   C. Blood from the urethral meatus
   D. Inability to void
   E. Dysuria after "straddle injury"

5. Anterior urethral "straddle injuries" occur most commonly in the:
   A. Bulbous urethra
   B. Pendulous urethra
   C. Fossa navicularis
   D. Membranous urethra

6. The most common cause of anterior urethral injuries are:
   A. Automobile accidents
   B. Falling off a ladder
   C. Iatrogenic
   D. Gunshot wound

THE FOLLOWING STATEMENT CONSISTS OF A STATEMENT AND A REASON. ANSWER BY USING THE FOLLOWING KEY:

   A. If both statement and reason are true and related as to cause and effect
   B. If both statement and reason are true but not related cause and effect
   C. If statement is true, but reason false
   D. If statement is false, but reason true

7. Blood and urinary extravasation into the perineum indicates bulbous urethral injury BECAUSE upward spread of the extravasation is limited by the urogenital diaphragm.

Genitourinary Injury

8. The optimum treatment for a patient with a bulbous urethral injury and who is voiding well would be:
   A. Foley catheter
   B. Suprapubic drainage
   C. Immediate repair
   D. C and A
   E. Observation

9. Bleeding secondary to injury of the urethra is generally from the:
   A. Dorsal artery of the penis
   B. The artery to the bulb
   C. Corpus cavernosum
   D. Corpus spongiosum

ANSWERS AND DISCUSSION

1. (D) Passage, or attempt at passage of a urethral catheter, in a patient such as this is to be condemned strongly. When blood is seen extruding from the urethral meatus, especially in a "straddle injury," one can assume that there has been a urethral injury and its extent should be evaluated by a retrograde urethrogram. Passage of a catheter would only aggravate the injury. Some would advise immediate suprapubic drainage and evaluation of the extent of injury at a later date, but this is a controversial issue at the time of this writing.

2. (A) If the patient does not void spontaneously, immediate repair soon after the injury would represent the optimum approach in a situation such as this. As was done in this case, the patient should be taken to the operating room and prepared for primary repair. This can be accomplished by debridement of the injured area with primary closure or end-to-end anastomosis of the urethra. Split-thickness skin grafts have been used in this area with success. If one wishes and one feels that the injury may be only a partial disruption of the urethra one can make a final attempt at passage of a catheter just prior to exploration, as was done here.

3. (E) Once Buck's fascia is opened by the injury, extravasated blood and urine is limited only by the boundaries of Colles' fascia, which extends into the perineum and scrotum and up onto the abdominal wall to continue with Scarpa's fascia, anteriorly. This is generally a much more severe injury with greater trauma to the area.

4. (C) The cardinal sign of injury to the anterior urethra is blood at the urethral meatus. Since the injury occurs below the area of the urethral sphincter, bleeding into the urethra from injury results in blood dribbling through the meatus. Injuries above the sphincteric area do not cause this sign since the sphincter prevents this and results in blood only in voiding.

5. (A) Since the bulbous portion of the urethra is in the perineum at the most accessible point of impact for this type of injury, this is the most commonly injured portion in this type of trauma.

6. (C) The most common anterior urethral injury is a perforating injury that may result when a metal sound is passed to dilate a stricture.

7. (A) The extravasation of blood and urine in rupture of the membranous urethra is almost always above the urogenital diaphragm, whereas, that from the bulb extends into the perineum and external genitalia. The firm attachments of the diaphragm limit the extent of this extravasation.

8. (E) If the patient can void well, and the perineal hematoma is not extensive, the injury can and should be observed. The blood generally will be reabsorbed and the tear in the urethra healed. Drainage should be performed if the hematoma becomes infected. Of course, follow-up examinations to make sure that the patient does not develop a urethral stricture are essential.

9. (D) The urethra is completely enveloped by the corpus spongiosum in its anterior portion, and bleeding will be secondary to associated rupture of this structure.

Genitourinary Injury   Case 16/ 83

CASE 16: 52-YEAR-OLD FEMALE WITH URINARY LEAKAGE AFTER ABDOMINAL SURGERY

HISTORY

A 52-year-old female underwent an abdominal perineal resection for carcinoma of the rectum. Dissection was made extremely difficult because of a large fibroid uterus, and because of this a total hysterectomy was performed simultaneously. The ureters had been dissected carefully during the procedure. On the 14th postoperative day, she noted urinary leakage from the perineal incision which persisted for several weeks. She was seen in consultation. An intravenous urogram revealed massive bilateral hydroretonephrosis, as well as a left ureteral fistula into the pelvis (Fig. 16.1). Preoperative intravenous urogram was within normal limits.

LABORATORY DATA

Hemoglobin 14gm%; hematocrit 33%; WBC 12,500 with a shift to the left. Blood urea nitrogen 20mg%. Urine analysis 30-40 WBC per high power field, otherwise normal. Urine culture showed more than 100,000 colonies of E. coli sensitive to most antibiotics tested.

PHYSICAL EXAMINATION

Blood pressure 130/70. Temperature normal 37°C. There was leakage of urine seen through a small opening in the perineum. The vagina was normal; and although there was induration in the pelvis, no masses could be palpated. A left lower quadrant colostomy was functioning well. There was no costovertebral angle tenderness. The remainder of the physical examination was normal.

QUESTIONS

1. Proper treatment at this point would be:
   A. Watchful waiting
   B. Bilateral nephrostomy
   C. Ureteral catheterization
   D. Ileal loop diversion

2. Proof of a minor fistula can be made by:
   A. Cystogram with indigo carmine
   B. Intravenous indigo carmine
   C. Retrograde ureteropyelogram
   D. All of the above

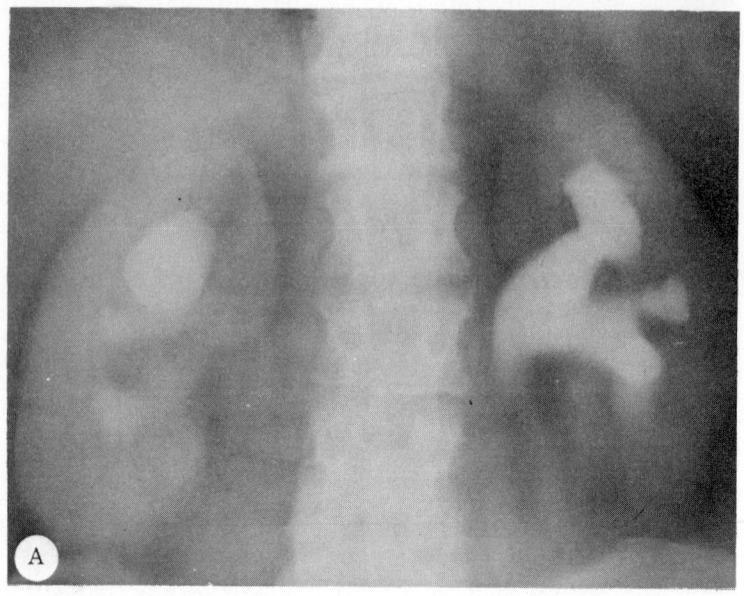
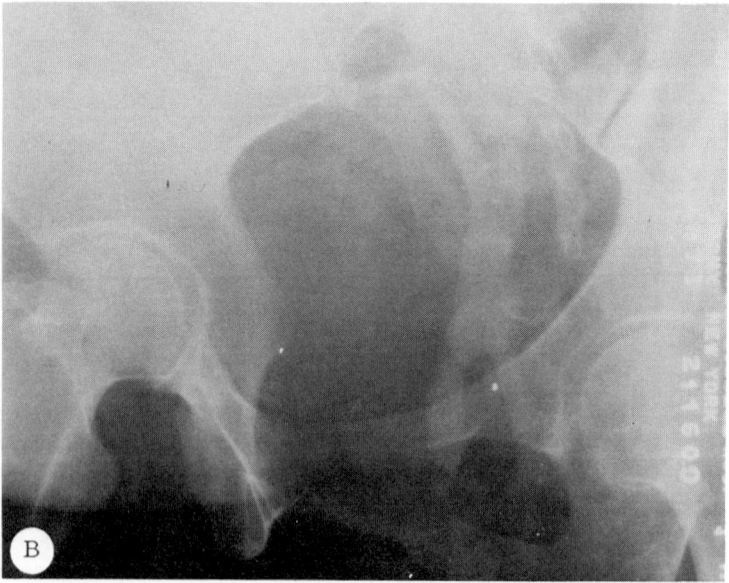

FIG. 16.1: Intravenous urogram showing bilateral hydroureteronephrosis (A) and a left ureteral fistula (B).

Genitourinary Injury

3. The diversion of choice for the surgically injured ureter is:
   A. Nephrostomy
   B. Cutaneous ureterostomy
   C. Ureterosigmoidostomy
   D. Ureterostomy in situ
   E. Nephrectomy

4. In gynecologic surgery, the zone where injury to the ureter is most likely to occur is:
   A. The iliac vessel
   B. The ovarian fossa
   C. The intraligamentary position of ureter
   D. The uterine artery
   E. All of the above

CLINICAL COURSE

A retrograde cystogram was performed and was normal with no evidence of extravasation. Bilateral retrograde ureteropyelogram showed a stricture at the junction of the middle and lower third of the right ureter and a fistula of the left ureter. A ureteral catheter was passed to the right renal pelvis, but none could be passed beyond the fistula on the left.

5. Proper treatment at this point would be:
   A. Left nephrostomy
   B. Left transureteroureterostomy
   C. Left ureteral reimplantation
   D. Left nephrectomy
   E. None of the above

A left nephrostomy was performed. The patient made an uneventful recovery. An intravenous urogram done three months after this showed a mild dilation on the right and a normal left collecting system (Fig. 16.2). She remains dry and free of infection. Five months after the left side was performed, the Gibbons catheter became obstructed and could not be replaced. A right ureteroneocystostomy was performed with a Boari bladder flap. She made an uneventful recovery following this. An intravenous urogram done two months after this is shown in Fig. 16.3. At this time, she was admitted for intestinal obstruction which responded to long tube drainage. She has done well following this and has been followed for eight months.

ANSWERS AND DISCUSSION

1. (C) In a situation such as this, ideal treatment would at least include temporary passage of ureteral catheter. This would

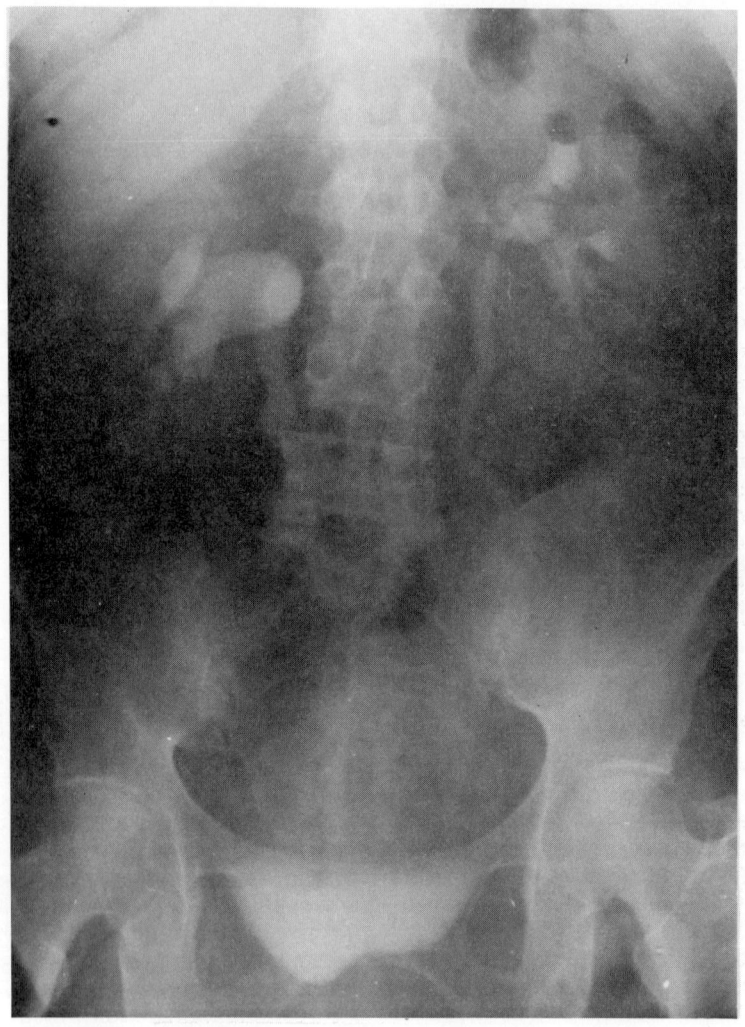

FIG. 16.2: Intravenous urogram with Gibbon's internal silastic stent on the right and nephrostomy on the left.

Genitourinary Injury

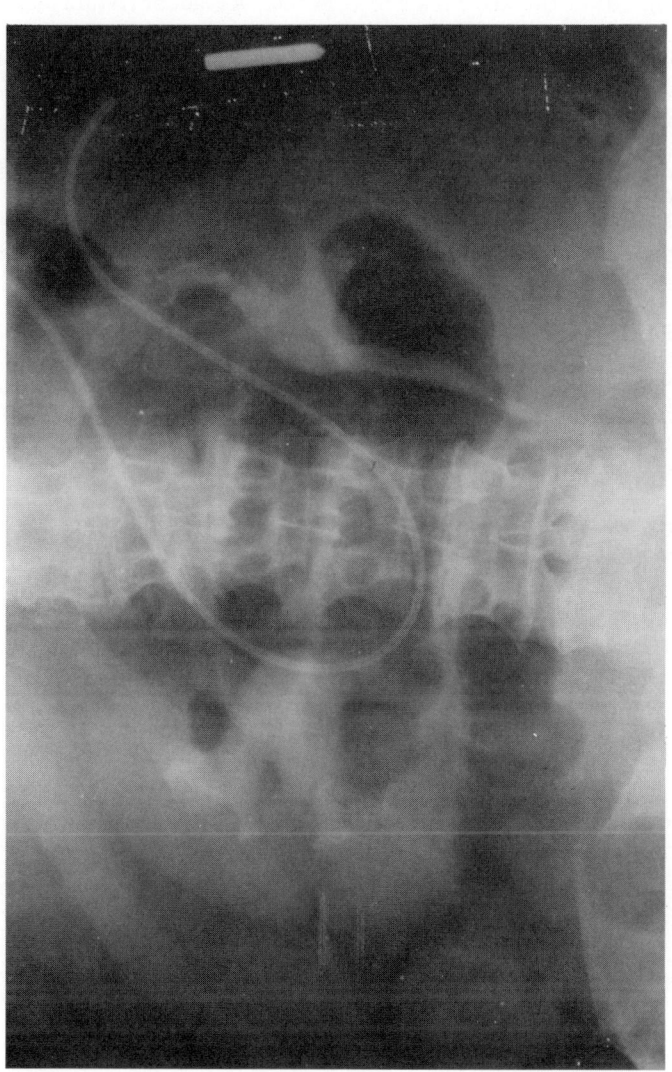

FIG. 16.3: Postoperative intravenous urogram.

allow for dilatation of any strictures that may be present and may even be curative for a small ureteral fistula. As shown, this was at least possible on the right side.

2. (D) All of the answers are correct. A bladder fistula would be demonstrable by retrograde cystogram and ureteral fistula by retrograde ureteropyelogram. Intravenous injection of indigo carmine would demonstrate a urinary fistula, but would not be definitive as to its location.

3. (A) Nephrostomy would be the procedure of choice if a ureteral catheter could not be passed to bypass obstruction. Nephrectomy may be indicated if the patient's prognosis is poor and there is a functioning, normal kidney on the opposite side.

4. (E) The ureter passes close to all of the structures mentioned and is likely to be injured at any one of these points. Careful dissection and identification of the ureter is essential to avoid injury. The ureter should be dissected with its surrounding connective tissue intact if later necrosis is to be avoided.

5. (A) As stated above, nephrostomy would be the procedure of choice.

CASE 17: 36-YEAR-OLD FEMALE WITH URINARY LEAKAGE FOLLOWING HYSTERECTOMY

HISTORY

A 36-year-old female had had her 4th delivery on January 13, 1965. She had a very difficult labor, and there was an unsuccessful attempt at midforceps delivery. She had a uterine rupture necessitating Cesarean hysterectomy. The bladder inadvertently was entered at the time of hysterectomy and closed with a double layer of chromic sutures. Soon after surgery, she began leaking urine from her vagina and continued to do so until she was seen in October, 1965. At that time, she was noted to have a tiny fistula; fulguration was attempted without success. Following this, the leaking increased in amount and on November 26, 1965, she underwent partial colpocleisis (Fig. 17.1). An urethral Foley was left indwelling for five days after which she voided very well; she has remained dry up to the time of this writing.

QUESTIONS

1. The most common site of posthysterectomy urinary fistula is:
    A. Vesicovaginal
    B. Right ureterovaginal
    C. Left ureterovaginal
    D. Urethrovaginal
    E. Ureterocutaneous fistula

2. You are called to the operating room because following a very difficult hysterectomy, urine is noted to be coming from a tear in the bladder. The first thing you would do is:
    A. Close the bladder in three layers
    B. Cytoscope the patient to see the exact location of the tear
    C. Do an I.V. urogram on the table
    D. Give indigo carmine intravenously

3. A vesicovaginal fistula which persists for five months after surgery that has not responded to fulguration is best treated by:
    A. Transvesical repair
    B. Transabdominal repair using an omental flap
    C. Transabdominal repair using a segment of ileum
    D. Transvaginal repair

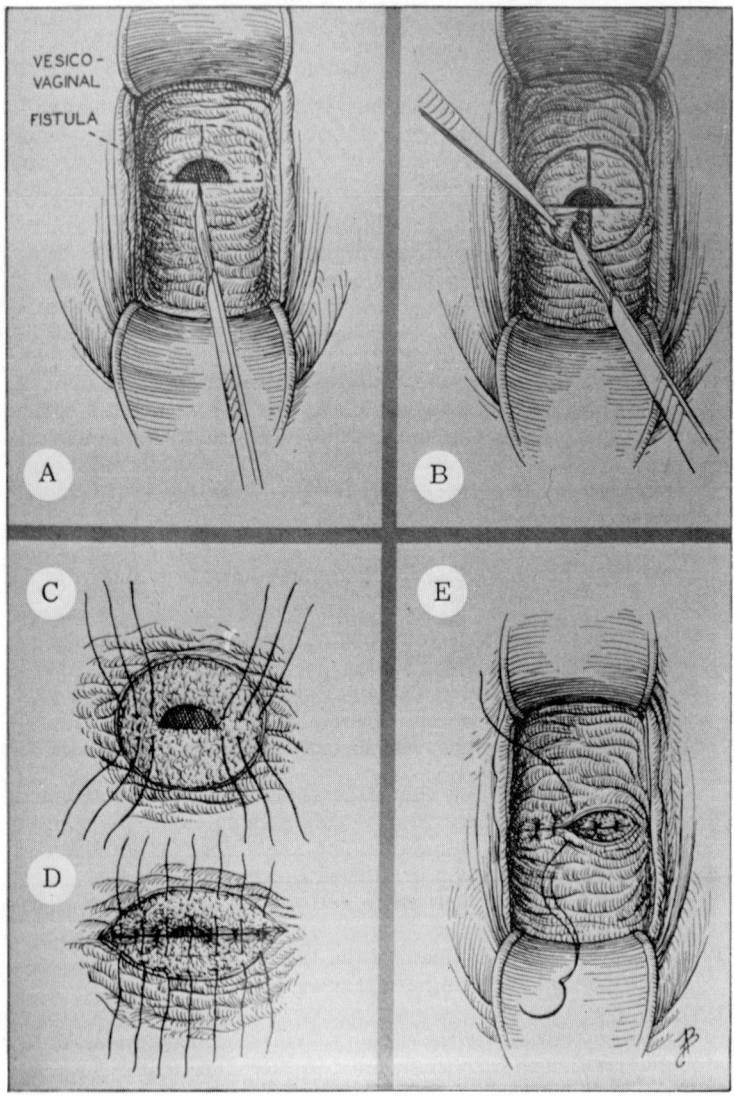

FIG. 17.1: Latzko procedure for vesicovaginal fistula (partial colpocleisis). From Greenhill JP: Surgical Gynecology, Year Book Medical Publishers, Chicago, 1952.

Genitourinary Injury   Case 17/ 91

4. In gynecologic surgery, the most likely area for injury to the ureter is where the ureter traverses:
   A. The iliac vessels
   B. The ovarian fossa
   C. The intraligamentary portion of ureter
   D. Close to the uterine artery
   E. All of the above

5. A 45-year-old female is seven days postvaginal hysterectomy and found to be leaking urine per vagina from a vesicovaginal fistula. Treatment of choice would be:
   A. Immediate surgery and closure of fistula
   B. Immediate fulguration of fistula
   C. Foley catheter drainage for three months
   D. Observation for three months and repair of fistula at that time if healing does not occur
   E. Suprapubic cystostomy

ANSWERS

1. (A) Vesicovaginal fistula is the most common postoperative urinary fistula seen. Invariably, they extend from the posterior wall of the bladder above the interureteric ridge into the vagina - generally at its apex along the suture line of closure of the vagina.

2. (D) After giving indigo carmine intravenously, one could then examine the interior of the bladder and note the blue dye coming from each ureteral orifice. This would signify that there is no associated ureteral injury. Once this has been established, the bladder then is closed carefully in three layers.

3. (D) As previously stated, most posthysterectomy vesicovaginal fistulae are from an area above the trigone to the apex of the vagina. These are best handled by the transvaginal approach. The technique of Latzko (see Fig. 17.1) has been advocated by most. Falk has repaired more than 100 such fistulae in this manner with excellent results.

4. (E) The ureter passes dangerously close to all the structures mentioned and can therefore be injured at the time of ligation of the ovarian vessels or the uterine artery, or as the ligaments are being divided. The proximity of the ureter must be remembered during the entire course of a hysterectomy. Identification of the ureter early in the dissection is essential.

5. (D) Immediate repair at seven days would be most hazardous and doomed to failure because of the severe inflammatory reaction going on at this time. Insertion of any foreign body, such as a Foley catheter or suprapubic tube, would only add to the inflammatory process and make later repair more difficult. The proper thing to do would be to observe her and repair the fistula in three months if it failed to close.

CHAPTER III

VESICOURETERAL REFLUX

INTRODUCTION

The normal ureterovesical junction allows the unidirectional flow of urine from kidney to bladder, preventing regurgitation into the kidney during the maximum pressure present during voiding. Incompetence of this valve mechanism gives rise to vesicoureteral reflux. Depending on its severity, and the presence or absence of infection, renal damage ensues. All agree that reflux is pathologic, but there is a wide divergence in methods of management.

Hutch has classified reflux as follows:

1. <u>Primary reflux</u>: This is secondary to trigonal weakness; Hutch believes that it improves with maturation. This is highly controversial.
2. <u>Obstructive reflux</u>
3. <u>Neurogenic reflux</u>: Reflux occurring in association with myelomeningocele and neurogenic bladder
4. <u>Inflammatory</u>: Reflux occurs commonly in the presence of infection.
5. <u>Congenital anomalies</u>: Ectopic ureters, duplication, etc.
6. <u>Iatrogenic</u>: Following surgery at the ureterovesical junction

The anatomy and physiology of the ureterovesical junction, as well as the theories of mechanisms of reflux are beyond the scope of this discussion and the reader is referred to standard textbooks of urology for this.

One cannot give a definite outline of the treatment of reflux, since it remains a point of disagreement, even among those expert in the field. In general, all children with mild forms of reflux, i.e., regurgitation only on voiding into normal appearing urinary tracts, can be managed conservatively. Those with marked amounts of reflux under low pressure with evidence of damage to the kidneys are managed surgically. The majority of patients seen with this disorder, however, fall somewhere in between these two extremes and require careful evaluation, several trials of medical management, and surgery only when conservative management fails.

The first case presented is the most commonly seen by the practicing urologist. These are easily managed conservatively by either intermittent short courses of antibiotics or long-term antibiotic therapy, as indicated in the individual situation. When this fails, as illustrated in Case #19, surgery is indicated. In the presence of normal ureters, success, i.e. absence of reflux and no evidence of complicating obstruction - can be expected in 90-95% of cases. When there is dilatation of the ureter, the success rate falls to 50-68%. About one-third of these children will continue to have infection, usually of a milder nature and without episodes of acute pyelonephritis. In severely damaged kidneys with no hope of return to some degree of function, total or partial nephrectomy is indicated.

Vesicoureteral Reflux

CASE 18: 6-YEAR-OLD GIRL WITH URINARY TRACT INFECTION

HISTORY

A 6-year-old girl was admitted to the hospital because of three episodes of documented urinary tract infections treated by her pediatrician. At the time of admission, urinalysis and culture were normal.

PHYSICAL EXAMINATION

Examination was entirely within normal limits.

LABORATORY DATA

An excretory urogram showed prompt bilateral excretion with normal upper urinary tracts. Retrograde cystogram performed at 15cm and 30cm of H_2O pressure above the bladder showed no evidence of vesicoureteral reflux. Voiding cystourethrogram revealed a normal urethra and evidence of reflux bilaterally (Fig. 18.1).

Urethral calibration with Bougie-a-boule showed the urethra to be 14F. Cystourethroscopy was normal.

CLINICAL COURSE

The urethra was dilated to 24F and the child was kept on nitrofurantoin for three months. Repeat cystogram and voiding urethrogram showed no evidence of reflux. Antibiotics were discontinued and the child has remained asymptomatic since that time. It is planned not to repeat the radiographic studies unless she develops another infection. Urinalysis and culture were performed every month initially, but now, at 3-month intervals.

QUESTIONS

1. Which of the following are considered etiologic factors in reflux?
    A. Bladder neck obstruction
    B. Urinary tract infection
    C. Short intravesical ureteral tunnel
    D. Paraureteral diverticulum
    E. All of the above

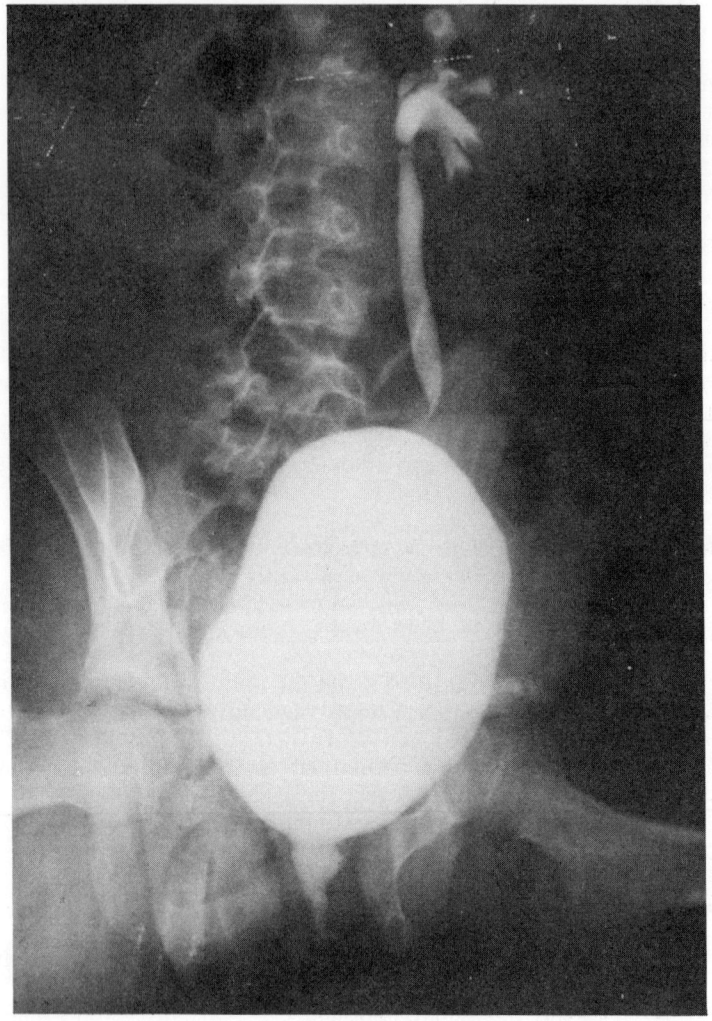

FIG. 18.1: Voiding cystourethrogram showing bilateral vesicoureteral reflux.

Vesicoureteral Reflux

2. Which of the following statements are false?
   A. The ureteral muscle extends downward and becomes the superficial trigone
   B. Waldeyer's sheath extends downward and becomes the deep trigone
   C. The superficial trigone inserts into the posterior urethra
   D. The deep trigone extends into the posterior urethra

3. Reflux is most commonly found at what age?
   A. At birth
   B. In the first year of life
   C. 1-3 years
   D. 3-6 years
   E. 6-12 years

4. What percentage of patients would you expect to remain well on conservative (nonoperative) management of reflux?
   A. 0-10%
   B. 20-30%
   C. 40-50%
   D. 70-75%
   E. 80-90%

5. The best indication for success of nonsurgical management would be:
   A. Absence of bladder trabeculation
   B. Configuration of the ureteral orifice
   C. Length of intravesical ureter
   D. Degree of dilatation of ureter
   E. Position of ureteral orifice on the trigone

6. Which of the following statements regarding "primary" reflux are false?
   A. Primary reflux is frequently familial
   B. Girls with primary reflux frequently have large bladder capacity and infrequent voiding
   C. A "golf hole" orifice is usually found
   D. Ureteral ectopia frequently is found
   E. It is always associated with bladder neck obstruction

7. If maturation is to cure the abnormality, at what age should reflux disappear?
   A. 4-6
   B. 6-8
   C. 8-10
   D. 10-12
   E. 14-16

8. What is the length of the intravesical ureter at birth?
   A. 0.5cm
   B. 1.0cm
   C. 1.5cm
   D. 2.0cm
   E. 2.5cm

ANSWERS AND DISCUSSION

1. (E) All the causes listed are considered etiologic factors in reflux. Bladder neck obstruction can be associated with reflux, and, if treated, the reflux frequently will disappear. Urinary infection alone, especially in children, frequently will cause reflux; and when treated, the reflux will frequently disappear as well. Ureteral competency is dependent on the length of the intravesical ureter, and a short tunnel will give rise to reflux. A diverticulum of the bladder through the ureteral hiatus causes shortening of the intravesical ureter and gives rise to reflux.

2. (D) The deep trigone, an extension of the Waldeyer's sheath, inserts into the bladder neck and does not go into the posterior urethra.

3. (D) King found that in 150 cases, nearly half were diagnosed between the age of 3 and 5.

4. (D) In a series of 323 refluxing ureteral units, King found that 51% stopped refluxing entirely, 20% remained well but reflux continued, and 4% remained well and refused further examination, a total of 75%.

5. (C) The length of the intravesical ureter appears to be the most important factor in ureterovesical junction competence. Even one that appears to be incompetent by the configuration of the orifice will not reflux if the intravesical length is adequate.

6. (E) Bladder neck obstruction may occasionally be found with reflux, but the latter factor may well be secondary rather than primary in nature.

7. (D) Hutch's theory of maturation proposes that the incompetent intramural ureter will, in the absence of infection, mature to normalcy by the time the child starts into puberty at the age of 10-12. This was based on the observation that at birth, the intravesical ureter was about 0.5cm long and

grew to approximately 1.3cm in the adult. Some question whether this will happen in the face of a grossly abnormal orifice.

8. (A)

REFERENCES

1. Tanagho EA and Pugh RCB: The anatomy, function of the ureterovesical junction. Brit J Urol 35:151-165, 1963.

2. Kelalis PP and King LR (eds.): Clinical Pediatric Urology, W.B. Saunders Company, Philadelphia, 1976, Chapter 11A, p. 342.

3. King LR, et al.: The case for nonsurgical management of vesicoureteral reflux. In: Current Controversies in Urology, W.B. Saunders Company, Philadelphia, 1972.

4. Hutch JA: Theory of maturation of the intravesical ureter. J Urol 86:534, 1961.

5. Lyon RP, Marshall S, and Tanagho EA: Theory of maturation: A critique. J Urol 103:795, 1970.

CASE 19: 9-YEAR-OLD GIRL WITH URINARY TRACT INFECTION

HISTORY

A 9-year-old white girl was seen because of urinary tract infections. She had been on nitrofurantoin for over two years and had repeated attacks of abdominal pain, fever, frequency, urgency, and positive urine cultures every 2-4 months.

PHYSICAL EXAMINATION

Initial examination was entirely within normal limits.

LABORATORY DATA

Routine lab data were normal. Excretory urogram showed prompt bilateral excretion and normal upper tracts. A retrograde cystogram showed bilateral high pressure reflux (Fig. 19.1A).

CLINICAL COURSE

She had another episode of infection while on suppressive therapy, which responded promptly to appropriate antibiotic therapy. A repeat retrograde cystogram six weeks later again showed bilateral high pressure reflux. She had another episode of acute infection three months later. A bilateral Leadbetter-Politano ureteral reimplantation was performed following this. Excretory urogram, retrograde cystogram, and voiding cystourethrogram were normal three months later, there being no evidence of reflux (Fig. 19.1B). The child has remained asymptomatic and the urine sterile in the absence of antimicrobial therapy.

QUESTIONS

1. Which of the following is not an indication for ureteral reimplantation for reflux?
    A. Renal scarring on ipsilateral side
    B. Stadium-shaped orifice
    C. "Golf hole" orifice
    D. Short intravesical ureter
    E. Dilatation of ureter

2. The most common complication of antireflux surgery is:
    A. Continued reflux
    B. **Obstruction**

Vesicoureteral Reflux   Case 19/ 101

    C. Continued pyelonephritis
    D. Renal atrophy

3. Contralateral ureteral reimplantation should be performed if:
    A. There is reflux contralaterally
    B. There is a short intravesical ureter, but no reflux is present
    C. There is a patulous orifice, but no reflux is present
    D. All of the above

4. In the presence of marked hydroureteronephrosis in a solitary kidney with reflux and azotemia the best method of preoperative preliminary drainage would be:
    A. Urethral catheter for several days
    B. Urethral catheter for as long as necessary to show improvement in the upper tract
    C. Suprapubic cystostomy
    D. Nephrostomy
    E. Cutaneous pyelostomy

5. Good results can be expected in which of the following operations for reflux:
    A. Leadbetter-Politano
    B. Pacquin
    C. Lich-Gregoir
    D. Glenn-Anderson
    E. All of the above

ANSWERS AND DISCUSSION

1. (B) All of the reasons given are considerations in determining whether surgery should be performed or not. They are not major reasons for surgery however, and this should be reviewed for children who continue to have infection or continue to show upper tract damage despite conservative therapy.

2. (B) Reflux following the usual methods of antireflux surgery is rather uncommon, occurring in less than 3% of patients with normal caliber ureter. Obstruction postoperatively would be a somewhat more common operative complication. Urinary tract infections may persist postoperatively, but are generally of a less severe nature.

3. (A) Fear of postoperative contralateral reflux should not be a reason for doing bilateral ureteral reimplantation.

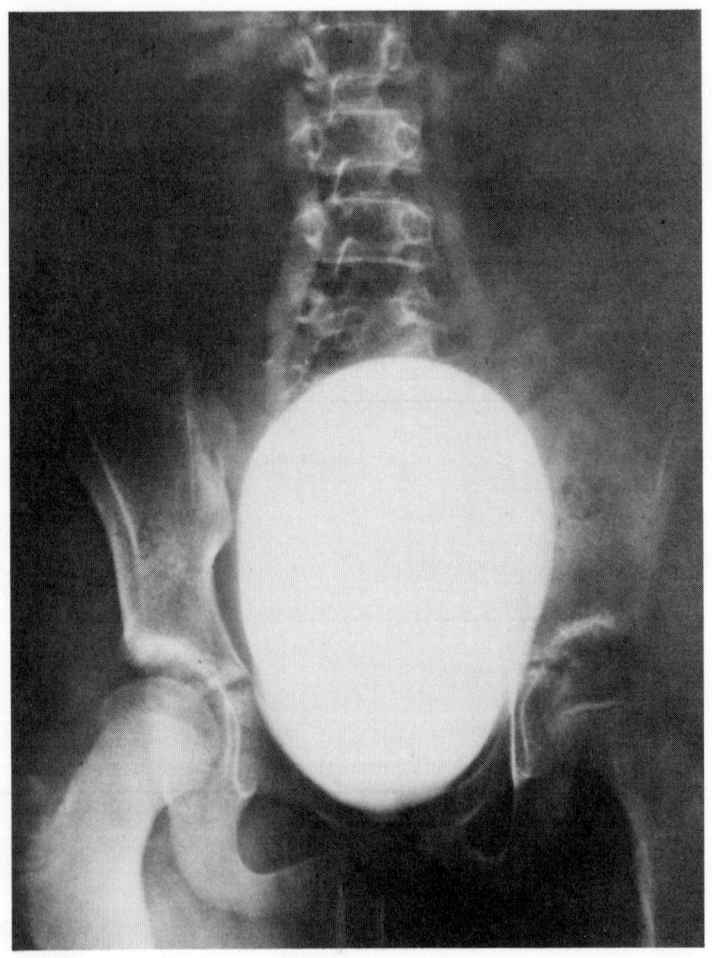

FIG. 19.1A: Retrograde cystogram showing a bilateral vesicoureteral reflux (see Fig. 19.1B).

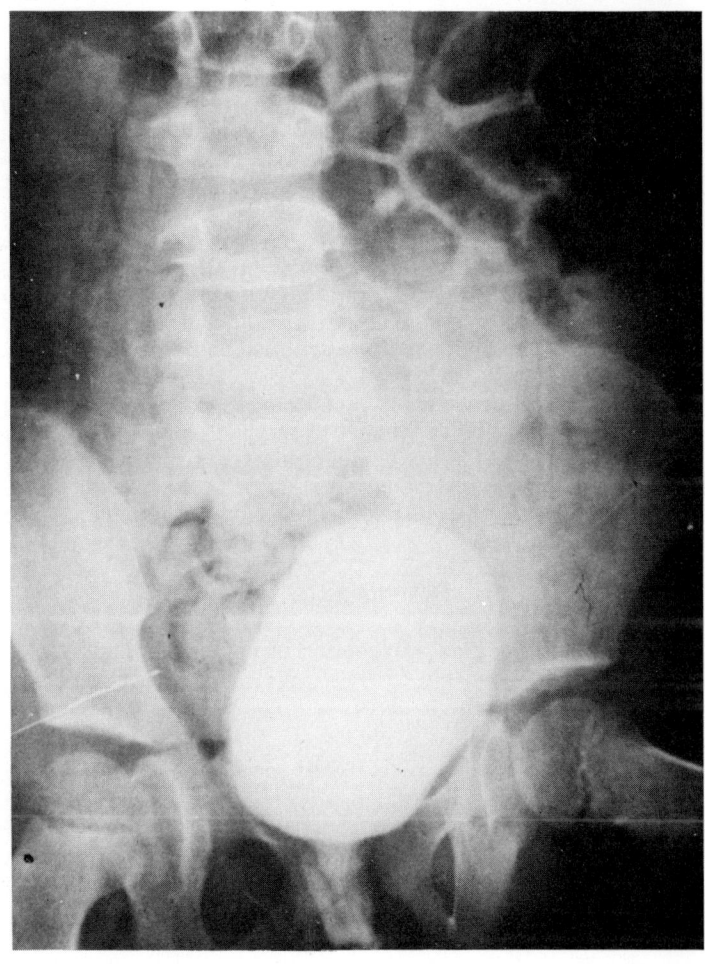

FIG. 19.1B: Retrograde cystogram showing no evidence of reflux.

Configuration of the orifice should not be used as an indication for surgery on the contralateral side if reflux cannot be demonstrated. Although it can occasionally be seen in the postoperative period following successful reimplantation, it is usually secondary to the inflammatory process of the trigone and will generally disappear with time.

4. (E) If there is marked dilation of the upper tract with diminished renal function and azotemia, it is best to provide temporary drainage prior to surgery on the ureterovesical junction. If this is to be prolonged, it would be best to do this by a "tubeless" technique such as cutaneous pyelostomy. Of course, this will require an operation for closure following successful reimplantation. If it is anticipated not to be of long duration, a nephrostomy may do. If there is minimal dilatation and azotemia, and only several days may be necessary for temporary drainage, and there is free drainage of the upper tract, a urethral catheter may suffice.

5. (E) All of the procedures mentioned are acceptable, and the type used would be dependent of the preference of the surgeon in regard to his experience and training. All have been reported as showing excellent results. The reader is referred to Kelalis' excellent description of the various techniques mentioned.

REFERENCE

1. Kelalis PP: Surgical correction of vesicoureteral reflux. In: Clinical Pediatric Urology, W. B. Saunders Company, Philadelphia, 1976, p. 366.

CASE 20: 2-MONTH-OLD CHILD WITH AN ABDOMINAL MASS

HISTORY

A 2-month-old child was admitted to the hospital because of a palpable abdominal mass on the left side. His birth history and growth and development were all normal. There was no history of urinary tract infections. There was no family history of genitourinary disorders.

PHYSICAL EXAMINATION

Blood pressure and pulse normal. There was a firm, movable mass in the left lower quadrant extending into the right side. The abdomen was mildly distended. Bowel sounds were normal.

LABORATORY DATA

Urinalysis, electrolytes, blood urea nitrogen, creatinine, and glucose were all within normal limits. A urine culture grew out E. coli sensitive to ampicillin with which the child was treated.

An intravenous urogram revealed nonvisualization at 3 minutes. On the 20-minute film a hydronephrotic pelvis was seen on the right side. On an 8-hour film the dilated pelvis, calyces and right ureter could be seen, but no contrast material was seen on the left, even up to 24 hours (Fig. 20.1A).

QUESTIONS

1. Differential diagnosis at this point would include:
    A. Bilateral primary megaureter
    B. Agenesis of left kidney
    C. Posterior urethral valves
    D. Ureterocele
    E. All of the above

2. The next step in differential diagnosis should be:
    A. Retrograde cystogram and voiding cystourethrogram
    B. Cystoscopy
    C. Infusion, intravenous urogram
    D. Angiogram
    E. Left renal exploration

A retrograde cystogram and voiding cystourethrogram were then performed; they revealed a markedly trabeculated bladder with evidence of massive reflux into the left, nonvisualized kidney as

106/ Case 20　　　　　　　　　　　　　　Vesicoureteral Reflux

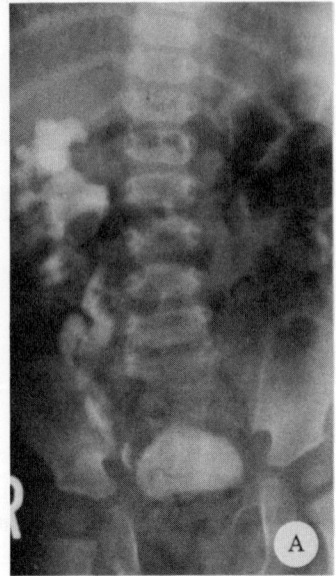 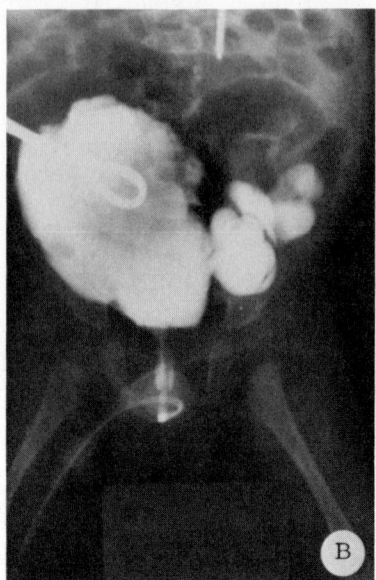

FIG. 20.1: (A) 8-hour intravenous urogram showing dilated right collecting system with no evidence of visualization on the left. (B) Voiding cystourethrogram showing posterior urethral valves and left vesicoureteral reflux.

well as posterior urethral valves (see Fig. 20.1B). An I_{131} Hippuran renogram showed only uptake on the right. A dilated ureter was seen on this side. There was no uptake on the left side.

3. Proper therapy at this point would be:
   A. Resection of valves only
   B. Resection of valves plus bilateral ureteral reimplantation
   C. Resection of valves plus left nephrectomy
   D. C+ right ureteral reimplantation

The child then underwent fulguration and resection of the posterior urethral valves, as well as a left nephroureterectomy. The kidney showed severe destruction of the cortex with only a few normal looking glomeruli. The rest of the parenchyma contained dilated tubules and fibrosis and, in addition, primitive ducts pathognomonic of dysplasia. He has been followed for one year and has been free of infection.

4. The incidence of reflux in posterior urethral valves is:
   A. Less than 10%

Vesicoureteral Reflux   Case 20/ 107

    B. 10-20%
    C. 20-30%
    D. 30-40%
    E. 40-50%

5. The presence of reflux associated with posterior urethral valves necessitates:
    A. Initial upper tract diversion
    B. Initial Foley catheter drainage
    C. Suprapubic catheter
    D. Ureteral reimplantation
    E. None of the above

6. Patients with reflux secondary to posterior urethral valves will require reimplantation in:
    A. 35% of cases
    B. 45% of cases
    C. 55% of cases
    D. 65% of cases
    E. 75% of cases

7. The radiographic findings pathognomonic of valves include:
    A. Dilatation of posterior urethra
    B. Narrow distal urethra
    C. Trabeculation of the bladder
    D. Widening of the bladder neck
    E. A & B

ANSWERS AND DISCUSSION

1. (E) Bilateral megaureter is a good possibility with severe damage of the left kidney, so much so that there is non-visualization. The kidney may also be congenitally absent. Posterior urethral valves should also enter the differential diagnosis with nonvisualization of the left kidney. A ureterocele can obstruct the bladder neck and thus cause bilateral obstruction.

2. (A)

3. (C)

4. (E) In the series of valves by Williams, et al., 44% of the patients had reflux preoperatively.

5. (E) Some believe that this requires immediate repair.

6. (E) Williams, however, has shown that 25% of these patients stopped refluxing spontaneously following relief of the obstructing valves. This has also been confirmed by Johnston. Reflux does not appear to effect the mortality of these children.

7. (E) The radiographic criteria used to diagnose posterior urethral valves have been: (a) Dilatation of the posterior urethra above the level of the obstructing valve in the posterior urethra. This dilatation should be present throughout the entire time of the voiding. There should also be seen a diminished stream beyond the area of obstruction.

REFERENCES

1. Kaplan GW: Chapter 106. In: Clinical Pediatric Urology, Kelalis PP and King LR (eds.), W.B. Saunders Company, Philadelphia, 1976.

2. Johnston JH and Kulatilake AE: The sequelae of posterior urethral valves. Brit J Urol 43:743-748, 1971.

3. Williams DI, et al.: Urethral valves. Brit J Urol 45:200-210, 1973.

CASE 21: 67-YEAR-OLD MALE WITH GROSS HEMATURIA

HISTORY

A 67-year-old man was admitted to the hospital because of gross total hematuria. He had nocturia 2-3 times nightly, but denied other urinary symptoms. He worked as a tailor and had never been exposed to chemicals. He had never smoked. He denied back pain, chills or fever.

PHYSICAL EXAMINATION

Blood pressure 140/70. Temperature normal. Chest and heart normal. There were no abdominal masses. Genitalia were normal. The prostate was slightly enlarged and benign.

LABORATORY DATA

Urinalysis 30-40 RBCs per high power field, otherwise normal. Hemoglobin 13.0gm%. Hematocrit 43%. Blood urea nitrogen 20mg%. Electrocardiogram and chest x-ray normal.

CLINICAL COURSE

An intravenous urogram showed prompt bilateral excretion with normal upper urinary tracts. The ureters were seen through their entire course and were normal. Cystoscopy revealed a 2cm papillary tumor along the ridge of the left ureter. The remainder of the bladder was free of tumor.

A transurethral resection of the tumor was carried out necessitating resection of almost the entire roof of the intramural ureter. A ureteral catheter was left indwelling for forty-eight hours. A retrograde cystogram done three months postoperatively showed vesicoureteral reflux into an undilated upper tract on the left side (Fig. 21.1).

Cytoscopies at 3-month intervals have shown no recurrent tumor. He remains asymptomatic and free of infection. Repeat intravenous urogram one year after surgery shows essentially no change. For the present, no treatment is planned for the reflux.

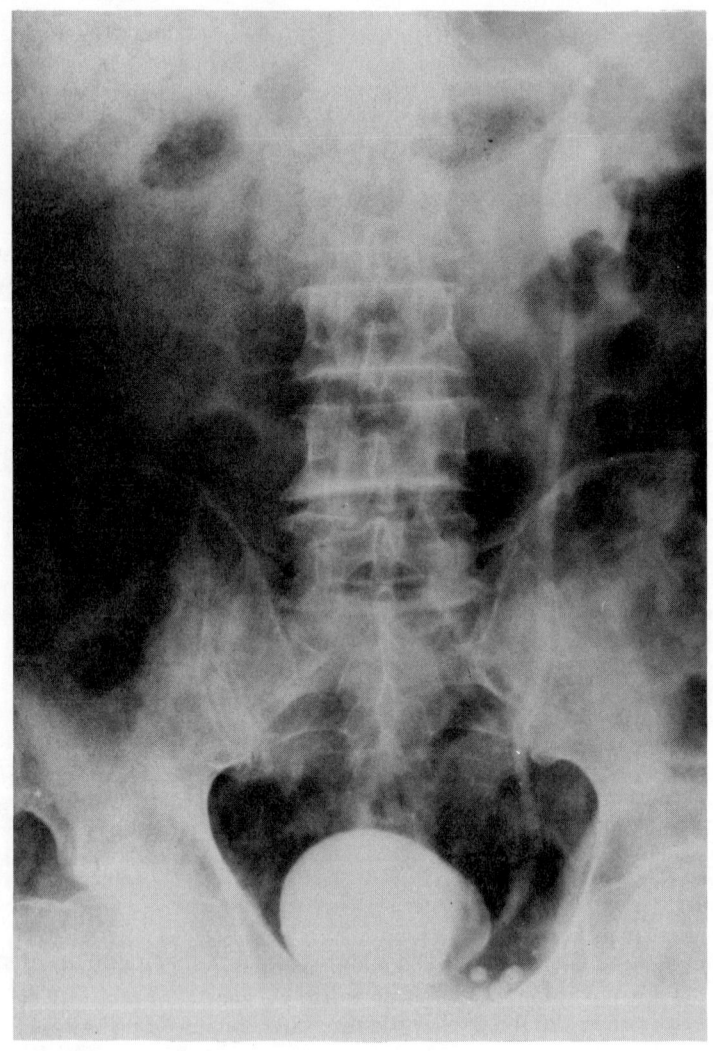

FIG. 21.1: Retrograde cystogram showing left vesicoureteral reflux.

CHAPTER IV

"NONSPECIFIC" INFECTIONS

INTRODUCTION

The "nonspecific" infections of the genitourinary tract are a group of diseases with similar manifestations caused by various microorganisms. These are distinguished from the "specific infections" of the urinary tract, such as tuberculosis or gonorrhea, which have characteristic clinical manifestations related to the specific infecting agent. Of the group of disorders under discussion, by far, the most common infecting bacteria are E. coli and other gram negative organisms. Streptococcus faecalis and staphylococcus are less common gram positive infecting agents. These bacteria can attack any of the genitourinary organs, causing symptoms of epididymitis, prostatitis, cystitis, etc.

The pathogenesis of genitourinary infections is generally believed to be of four varieties. Ascending infection is probably the most common, with invasion of organisms of the lower urinary tract establishing infection and ascending to cause cystitis, pyelonephritis, etc. Hematogenous infection is probably less common than previously believed. In this type, there is metastatic spread from infection in another part of the body to the urinary tract. Perinephric abscess in drug addicts (see Case 24) is an illustration of this type of infection. Lymphogenous spread from inflammatory disease of other pelvic organs is another possible mode of pathogenesis. Direct extension to the genitourinary tract by appendiceal abscess, diverticulitis, or regional enteritis is not uncommonly seen presenting as a urologic problem (see Case 26).

CASE 22: 72-YEAR-OLD FEMALE WITH NAUSEA AND VOMITING

HISTORY

A 72-year-old female was admitted because of nausea and vomiting of one week's duration. She also complained of severe weakness. She had an 8-year history of recurrent bladder tumor, and had had four transurethral resections for bladder tumor. These were all reported Grade I transitional cell carcinoma, with no evidence of invasion of the bladder wall. For all the past two years prior to admission, her BUN ranged from 30 to 40mg%. Her past history was otherwise negative.

PHYSICAL EXAMINATION

Blood pressure 170/90, pulse 86 regular. She was a small, frail woman in no distress. There were diffuse rhonchi in the chest. There were no abdominal masses. Pelvic examination was normal. There was no CVA tenderness.

LABORATORY DATA

Hemoglobin 9.8gm%, hematocrit 37%. Blood urea nitrogen on admission was 85mg%, creatinine 8.2mg%. Urinalysis was normal, and a urine culture showed no growth. A renal scan revealed decreased function bilaterally with small, contracted kidneys.

HOSPITAL COURSE

She was treated with hydration, and her urinary output was good. The blood urea nitrogen fell to 42mg%, and the creatinine to 3.5 mg%. The nausea, vomiting and weakness improved. An infusion intravenous urogram revealed small, contracted kidneys bilaterally (Fig. 22.1). Cystoscopy showed no evidence of recurrent tumor. She was discharged, and renal function has remained stable for four months following the episode.

QUESTIONS

1. The changes in the kidney thought to be most specific for bacterial damage are:
    A. Cortical scarring
    B. Destruction of tubules
    C. Glomerular scarring
    D. Retraction of papilla
    E. A & D

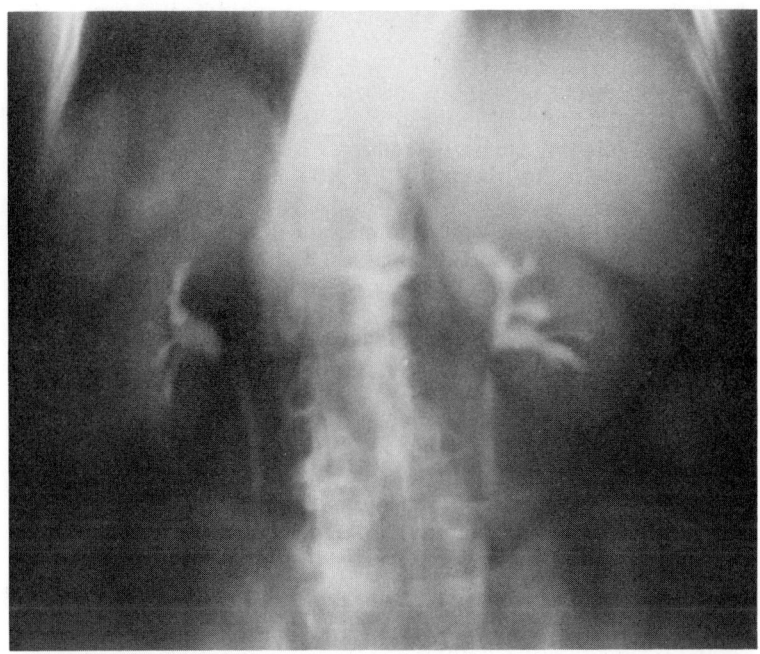

FIG. 22.1: Infusion intravenous urogram showing small, contracted kidneys bilaterally.

2. Which of the following are pathognomonic of chronic pyelonephritis?
   A. Positive renal biopsy
   B. White blood cell casts
   C. Typical pyelographic changes
   D. Red blood cell casts
   E. None of the above

3. The characteristic renal function abnormality of early chronic pyelonephritis is:
   A. Decreased renal blood flow
   B. Poor concentrating ability and normal glomerular function
   C. Poor concentrating ability and decreased glomerular function
   D. Normal concentrating ability and decreased glomerular function
   E. None of the above

4. Which of the following is not a radiographic finding in chronic pyelonephritis?
   A. Small kidney
   B. Cortical scarring
   C. "Clubbing" of calyces
   D. Edema of pelvic mucosa
   E. None of the above

5. Which of the following can mimic the clinical and radiographic finding of chronic pyelonephritis?
   A. Sickle cell anemia
   B. Potassium depletion
   C. Phenacetin ingestion
   D. Diabetes mellitus
   E. All of the above

ANSWERS AND DISCUSSION

1. (E) The change in the kidney believed to be most specific for damage secondary to bacterial infection is a broad scar of the renal parenchyma associated with retraction of the corresponding renal papilla. This has been established both clinically as well as pathologically.

2. (E) Although all of the findings may be associated with chronic pyelonephritis, none are definitely diagnostic, and the diagnosis must be made not on one clinical finding, but on the correlation of many findings. The presence of a history of urinary tract infections, bacteruria, white cell casts in the urine, the typical pyelographic changes, as well as functional changes all would have to be present to make a definitive diagnosis.

3. (B) The tubular portion of the kidney is apt to suffer the greatest degree of damage in chronic pyelonephritis, and, this being the case, there is more interference with tubular transport system than with glomerular filtration. Therefore, one is likely to find a poor concentrating ability to be present with fairly normal glomerular function.

4. (D) The typical radiographic findings, as described by Hodson, are small, contracted kidneys, cortical scarring and loss of cupping of the calyces secondary to retraction of the calyx. Edema of the pelvic mucosa is a finding sometimes seen radiographically in acute pyelonephritis.

5. (E) All of those listed, plus many others, including obstruction and acute tubular necrosis, are capable of producing

significant interstitial changes in the kidney, and mimic chronic pyelonephritis both clinically, as well as radiographically.

REFERENCES

1. Freedman LR: Urinary tract infection, pyelonephritis and other forms of chronic interstitial nephritis, Chapter 18. In: Diseases of the Kidney, Strauss MB and Welt LG (eds.), Little, Brown and Co., Boston, 1971, p. 668.

2. Hodson CJ: The radiologic contribution toward the diagnosis of chronic pyelonephritis. Radiology 88:857, 1967.

CASE 23: 25-YEAR-OLD FEMALE WITH DYSURIA AND FEVER

HISTORY

This 25-year-old female was well until approximately ten days prior to admission to the hospital, when she developed dysuria associated with high fever. She was seen in the emergency room, where a urinary infection secondary to gram negative rods was discovered. She was placed on ampicillin, but her temperature remained 101°, and she was admitted to the hospital. She complained of left flank and left upper quadrant pain, but the dysuria subsided after starting ampicillin. Her temperature on admission was 104°, and she appeared acutely ill. She gave a strong family history of polycystic renal disease in her father, paternal grandmother, and paternal aunt.

PHYSICAL EXAMINATION

The patient appeared ill and in distress because of left upper quadrant and flank pain. Blood pressure was 110/70, temperature 104°, pulse 105 per minute. There was marked left CVA and left upper quadrant tenderness, with some fullness in the left upper quadrant, but no definite masses palpable. The remainder of the physical examination was unremarkable.

LABORATORY DATA

WBC 8700; normal differential. Hematocrit 39%; chest x-ray normal; urine 3-5 WBC/high/power/field; blood urea nitrogen 10mg%; creatinine 0.9mg%; urine cultures and multiple blood cultures showed no growth. The remainder of the chemical profile was normal.

An intravenous urogram revealed bilateral cysts, the largest of which was in the left lower pole (Fig. 23.1). This was consistent with polycystic kidney disease.

CLINICAL COURSE

She continued to run a febrile course spiking to $101-103^O$ daily, and, in spite of antibiotic therapy, continued to have marked tenderness on the left side. Therefore, renal exploration was carried out. A large, infected, thick-walled cyst was found at the lower pole of the left kidney. This was biopsied, and a diagnosis of xanthogranulomatous pyelonephritis was found. The abscess was drained, and she made an uneventful recovery. She has been followed for $3\frac{1}{4}$ years, and renal function is stable, and there has been little change in the intravenous urogram.

"Nonspecific" Infections

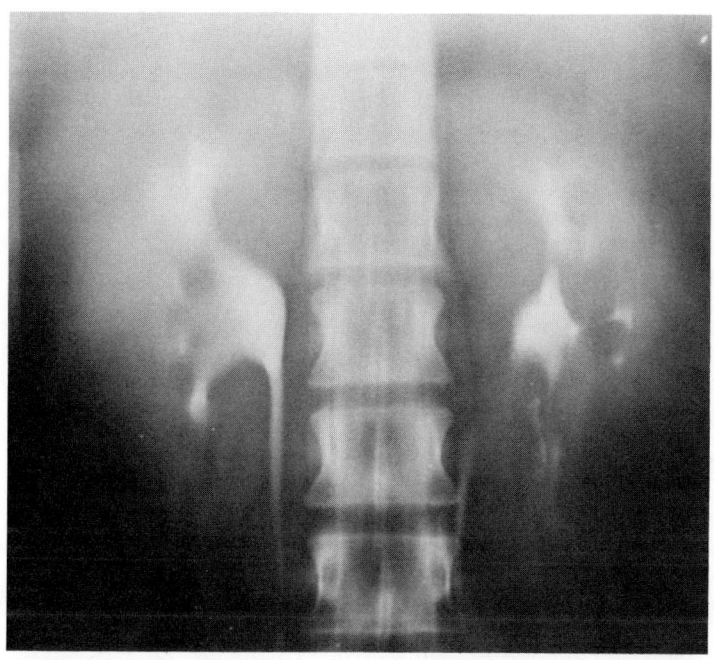

FIG. 23.1: Intravenous urogram (with tomography) showing bilateral renal cyst, the largest being in the left lower pole.

QUESTIONS

1. The following are all characteristic of xanthogranulomatous pyelonephritis, except:
   A. Chronic renal parenchymal infection with abscess formation
   B. Associated calculus disease
   C. Granuloma formation
   D. Caseation
   E. Giant foam cells

(T)RUE OR (F)ALSE:

2. A nonfunctioning kidney on intravenous urography occurs in the majority of patients with xanthogranulomatous pyelonephritis.

3. Nephrolithiasis is a common accompaniment of xanthogranulomatous pyelonephritis.

4. Xanthogranulomatous pyelonephritis can rarely be confused with renal cell carcinoma.

5. Treatment of xanthogranulomatous pyelonephritis always is by nephrectomy.

6. Lipid-laden histocytes are commonly adjacent to granuloma of the xanthogranulomatous pyelonephritis.

ANSWERS AND DISCUSSION

1. (D) Xanthogranulomatous pyelonephritis has been defined as an atypical form of severe, chronic renal parenchymal infection, characterized by variable destruction of renal parenchyma, and usually associated with calculi and granulomas with or without abscess formation.

2. (T) In the review of xanthogranulomatous pyelonephritis reported by Noyes and Palubinskos, 85% of the cases were associated with a nonfunctioning kidney, and 15% presented with a functioning kidney with evidence of a renal mass.

3. (T) Nephrolithiasis, commonly, is associated with xanthogranulomatous pyelonephritis. In our series,[2] 15 of the 27 kidneys showed evidence of calculi. In other series, the incidence ranges from 22-80%.

4. (F) Clinically, the two entities can easily be confused, and frequently are. A mass present on intravenous urography can easily be interpreted as either carcinoma or granulomatous disease. The angiographic appearance of xanthogranulomas varies with the extent of the disease. The avascular mass produced by this disease can be confused with an avascular pattern of carcinoma. Even histologically, the large, foamy histocytes, on superficial inspection, can easily be interpreted as renal cell carcinoma cells.

5. (F) Although nephrectomy is frequently performed because of the factors mentioned above, this is not absolutely necessary. In our series of 27 cases, two were diagnosed by biopsy, and one by partial nephrectomy. All three kidneys continue to function well, with better than a 2-year follow-up in all three cases.[2]

6. (T) The characteristic microscopic finding in this disorder is abscess formation. The abscesses are usually multiple,

with central necrosis and chronic inflammatory cells, and the lipid-laden histocytes are commonly seen in the adjacent area.

REFERENCES

1. Noyes WE and Palubinskas AJ: Xanthogranulomatous pyelonephritis. J Urol 101:132-136, 1969.

2. Tolia BP, et al.: Xanthogranulomatous Pyelonephritis: A Critical Analysis of 27 Cases with Unusual Presentation in Four (to be published).

3. Anhalt MA, Cawood CD, and Scott R, Jr: Xanthogranulomatous pyelonephritis: A comprehensive review with report of four additional cases. J Urol 105:10, 1971.

CASE 24: 27-YEAR-OLD MALE WITH RIGHT UPPER QUADRANT PAIN

HISTORY

A 27-year-old drug addict was admitted to the hospital in August, 1970. Four weeks prior to admission, he experienced right upper quadrant pain and anorexia, followed by a 25-pound weight loss. Two weeks prior to admission, he noted a mass in the right upper quadrant, which had been increasing in size. For three days prior to admission, he had fever and chills. He denied dysuria, frequency, nocturia, or difficulty in voiding. There was no past history of renal disease or urinary calculi.

PHYSICAL EXAMINATION

A thin, cachectic male with abdominal discomfort. Temperature was 102.4°; blood pressure 120/70; pulse 120 per minute. There was a visible mass in the abdomen, 8 x 14cm, which was exquisitely tender. This was noted to be separate from the liver. There was minimal costovertebral angle tenderness. Remainder of the physical examination was normal.

LABORATORY DATA

Hemoglobin 11.2gm%; WBC 18,300; 70% polys; urinalysis showed many WBCs and 1-2 RBCs; urine culture showed no growth. Blood urea nitrogen 10mg%; electrolytes normal; chest x-ray normal. Intravenous urogram showed a right upper quadrant mass, a large kidney with distortion of calyces (Fig. 24.1). An arteriogram was performed, revealing abnormal vasculature in the area of the mass.

CLINICAL COURSE

The patient was placed on ampicillin and kanamycin and I.V. fluids. Exploration of the right flank was performed two days after admission, and a perinephric abscess was found, culture of which grew out Staphylococcus aureus coagulase positive. A nephrectomy was performed, and the patient made an uneventful recovery. The kidney was found to be almost totally destroyed by the inflammatory process.

QUESTIONS

1. Perinephric abscess is generally found:
   A. Beneath the renal capsule and outside the renal parenchyma

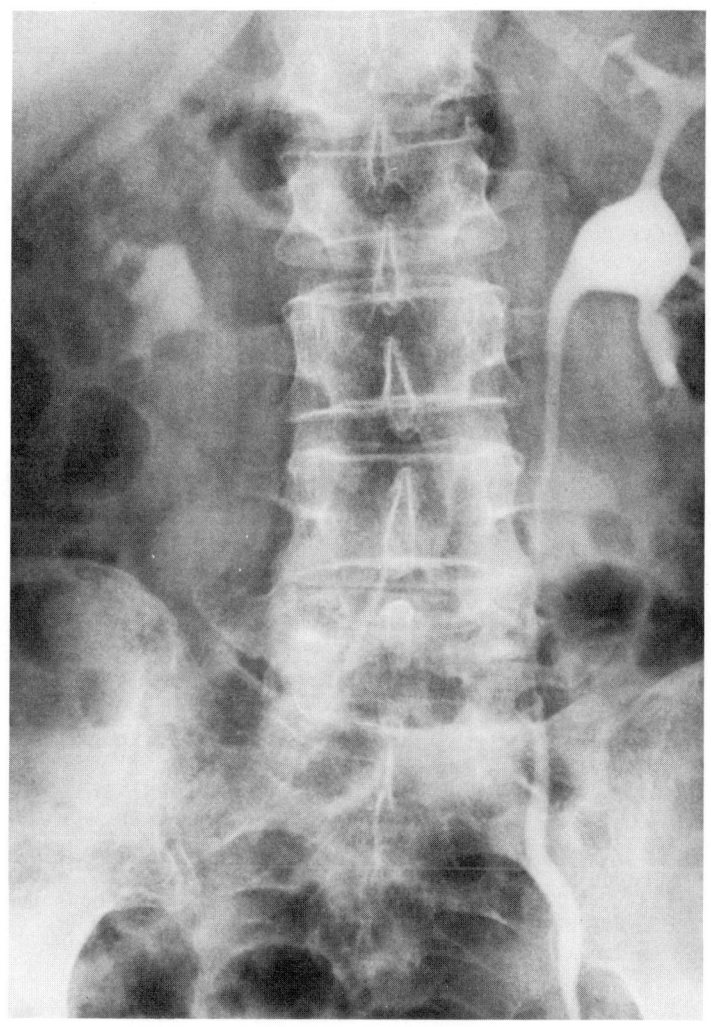

FIG. 24.1: Intravenous urogram. There is distortion of the calyces on the right.

Case 24 — "Nonspecific" Infections

   B. Between the renal capsule and Gerota's fascia
   C. Outside Gerota's fascia
   D. From the collecting system into the renal parenchyma

2. Which of the following are not radiographic signs of perinephric abscess?
   A. Flank mass
   B. Obliteration of psoas margin
   C. Free air in the retroperitoneum
   D. Nonvisualization of kidney
   E. Scoliosis of the spine

3. The etiology of perinephric abscess is generally:
   A. Extension from cortical abscess in chronic pyelonephritis
   B. Calculous pyonephrosis
   C. Metastatic abscess from skin
   D. All of the above

EACH OF THE FOLLOWING STATEMENTS CONSISTS OF A STATEMENT AND A REASON. ANSWER BY USING THE FOLLOWING KEY:

   A. If both statement and reason are true and related, cause and effect
   B. If both statement and reason are true but not related, cause and effect
   C. If statement is true, but the reason false
   D. If statement is false, but reason is true
   E. If both statement and reason are false

4. A perinephric abscess may present just above the iliac crest posterolaterally BECAUSE the space between Gerota's fascia and the kidney expands inferiorly to this area.

5. Ureteral compression is rare in perinephric abscess BECAUSE the ureter does not lie within the fascial planes of the abscess.

6. Inspiratory and expiratory films on the excretory urogram are helpful in diagnosis of perinephric abscess BECAUSE the diaphragm will not move with this disease.

ANSWERS AND DISCUSSION

1. (B) Perinephric abscess can be secondary to a renal carbuncle or severe staphylococcal infection of the kidney, or

an advanced chronic pyelonephritis with or without renal calculus. It is an infection of the tissue between the renal capsule and Gerota's fascia. The abscess can become quite large, sometimes pointing posteriorly over the iliac crest, or even in the anterior thigh. Today, they are most commonly seen in drug addicts secondary to metastatic staphylococcal infection from contaminated needles or cutaneous infections.

If the abscess can be found in its early stages, prior to destructive changes in the kidney, incision and drainage is the treatment of choice. As in the case presented here, however, there is little to be gained by leaving a totally destroyed, badly infected kidney.

2. (D) Flank mass is typical in perinephric abscess and, as in this case, may be the presenting symptom. Edema, invariably present, obliterates the psoas and, sometimes, the renal margins. Gas-forming gram negative organisms are common etiologic agents, and can show typical spotty deposits of gas in the retroperitoneum. Scoliosis of the spine with its concavity to the affected side is a classical sign of perinephric abscess. Nonvisualization of the kidney is not commonly found, although the kidney is usually severely damaged.

3. (D) As stated previously, etiology can be by direct extension or metastatic. Extension of chronic pyelonephritis in a diabetic is not an uncommon situation. Here, generally, the organism would be a gram negative one, and may be gas-forming. Calculous pyenephrosis may extend into the perinephric space, and cause abscess formation as well.

4. (A) Perinephric abscess may present in Petit's triangle. This is a rare situation, but may occur specifically for the reason given. Perinephric abscess has been seen to extend down the entire retroperitoneum and into the thigh, following the course of the psoas muscle. Rarely, too, it can cross the spine within the perirenal fascia and involve the other side.

5. (E) Hydronephrosis may develop from ureteral compression, since the abscess generally surrounds the ureter beneath Gerota's fascia. Even after the abscess is drained, ureteral compression may develop with scarring and, if nephrectomy is not indicated, follow-up excretory urograms must be obtained to be certain that this has not occurred. This is usually done in 2-3 months.

6. (C) Lack of movement of the kidney on inspiratory and expiratory films is strongly suggestive of a perinephric inflammatory process, and can be a very helpful diagnosis. The diaphragm may be elevated and fixed as well, if the abscess extends superiorly in this direction.

REFERENCE

1. Salvatierra O, Jr, Bricklew WB, and Morrow H: Perinephric abscess: A report of 71 cases. J Urol 98:296-306, 1967.

CASE 25: 57-YEAR-OLD FEMALE WITH GROSS HEMATURIA

HISTORY

A 57-year-old white female was admitted to the hospital with a history of intermittent, gross, painless hematuria. She denied history of renal stones, fever, or dysuria. She had had a similar episode of hematuria 19 years ago, but did not seek medical aid at that time. She had a history of hypertension. There was no history of analgesic abuse.

PHYSICAL EXAMINATION

A blood pressure of 200/120, but otherwise unremarkable.

LABORATORY DATA

Urinalysis revealed many RBCs, only occasional WBCs. Urine culture showed no growth. Fasting blood sugar 354mg%, blood urea nitrogen 18mg%, creatinine 1mg%.

CLINICAL COURSE

An intravenous urogram showed abnormal right kidney with very poor function on the left. Cystoscopy was performed, and the bladder was normal. A left retrograde pyelogram (Fig. 25.1) revealed caliectasis of the lower pole, and urinary sediment had tissue that, on section, was consistent with papillary necrosis. She was treated conservatively, and the bleeding gradually subsided. Her diabetes responded to oral hypoglycemics and diet, and the urine remains sterile.

QUESTIONS

1. Which of the following are not etiologic factors in papillary necrosis?
    A. Diabetes
    B. Chronic pyelonephritis
    C. Sickle cell trait
    D. Phenacetin ingestion
    E. None of the above

2. The typical pyelographic findings in papillary necrosis are:
    A. "Ring sign" in the area of the renal papilla
    B. Filling defect in pelvis
    C. "Inverted flask sign" in area of papilla
    D. All of the above
    E. None of the above

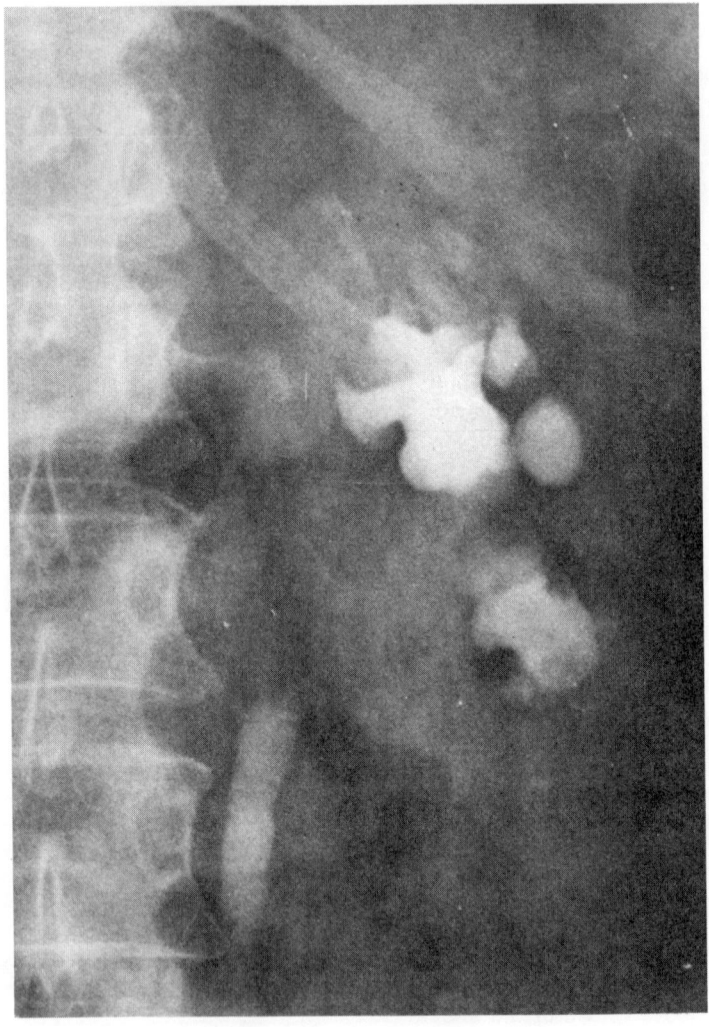

FIG. 25.1: Retrograde pyelogram showing caliectasis, consistent with papillary necrosis.

"Nonspecific" Infections   Case 25/ 127

3. Calculi following papillary necrosis are characterized by:
    A. "Jackstone" type
    B. "Waxy" appearance
    C. Radiolucent center and radiopaque periphery
    D. Attachment to papilla

4. Nitrofurantoin has which of the following side-effects?
    A. Peripheral neuropathy
    B. Hemolytic anemia
    C. Jaundice
    D. Pneumonia
    E. All of the above

5. Cephalexin is:
    A. Penicillinase sensitive
    B. Penicillinase resistant
    C. Ineffective against gram positive cocci
    D. Poorly absorbed from GI tract
    E. None of the above

REGARDING THE FOLLOWING NUMBERED DRUGS, MATCH EACH ONE WITH ITS LETTERED DEGREE OF EFFECTIVENESS IN VIVO AGAINST GRAM NEGATIVE PATHOGENS.

6. ___Nitrofurantoin   A. Most effective
7. ___Colistin   B. Second
8. ___Cephalothin   C. Third
9. ___Chloramphenicol   D. Fourth
10. ___Ampicillin   E. Fifth

ANSWERS AND DISCUSSION

1. (E) Papillary necrosis is a common type of renal inflammatory disease. At one time, it was thought to be confined to diabetics, but it has been seen in pyelonephritis without diabetes as well. Excessive phenacetin ingestion and sickle cell trait are other known causes of papillary necrosis.

    The disease can be bilateral and, in these cases, it is generally severe. Oliguria, uremia, and sepsis may occur rapidly. The kidney may heal, and the necrotic papilla may serve as the nucleus for calculus formation. Rarely, nephrectomy is required for intractable bleeding or infection with destruction of the kidney.

2. (D) All of the listed signs may be found, and have been described very nicely by Harrow. The reader is referred to

this article. The typical cavities seen in the totally destroyed papilla are late signs of papillary necrosis.

3. (C) Calculus formation, as a late complication of papillary necrosis occurs, and is characterized by, irregular calcified bodies with radiolucent centers, which represents both the sloughed papilla which has not been excreted and deposition of calcium on itself.

4. (E) All of the side-effects listed have been ascribed to nitrofurantoin.

5. (B) Cephalexin is a penicillinase-resistant antibiotic, and effective against penicillinase-producing organisms.

6. (E) Seneca, et al., evaluated the efficacy of various drugs
7. (B) in gram negative human pathogens, and found the
8. (D) relative effects as shown in these answers. Although
9. (C) colistin was found to affect more of the 100-gram
10. (A) negative rods tested in vitro, the in vivo effect of ampicillin was found to be almost 90%, as compared to 72% for colistin.

REFERENCES

1. Harrow BR, et al.: Roentgenologic demonstration of renal papillary necrosis in sickle cell trait. New Eng J Med 268: 969-976, 1963.

2. Harrow BR: Renal papillary necrosis: A critique of pathogenesis. J Urol 97:203, 1967.

3. Seneca H, Peer P, and Warren B: Efficacy of drugs in gram negative urinary pathogens. J Urol 99:337, 1968.

CASE 26: 64-YEAR-OLD MALE WITH FREQUENCY, DYSURIA AND NOCTURIA

HISTORY

A 64-year-old male was seen because of frequency of urination, dysuria, nocturia 2 to 3 times, and gross terminal hematuria. This had been present for the past 5 to 6 weeks. There was no history of flank pain, chills, or fever. He denied any changes in bowel habits, diarrhea, bloody stool, or abdominal pain.

QUESTIONS

1. The significance of gross terminal hematuria is:
   A. Bleeding is distal to the external sphincter
   B. Bleeding is secondary to a lesion in the fossa navicularis at the tip of the penis
   C. Bleeding may be secondary to a bladder lesion
   D. Bleeding cannot be from the bladder
   E. Upper urinary tract pathology is definitely ruled out

PHYSICAL EXAMINATION

The blood pressure was 170/100. Heart and chest were normal. The abdomen was soft, flat, and nontender. There were no masses palpable, and bowel sounds were normal. Rectal examination was unremarkable.

LABORATORY DATA

Normal hemogram. Urinalysis showed 1+ albumin and many WBCs per high power field. Urine culture revealed more than 100,000 colonies of E. coli per ml of urine, sensitive to most antibiotics tested. An intravenous urogram revealed prompt bilateral excretion with normal upper tracts. The excretory cystogram was normal.

CLINICAL COURSE

Cystoscopy was performed and there was no evidence of obstruction. On the superior wall of the bladder was an elevated, reddened, edematous area approximately 2 cm in diameter, raising the suspicion of an extrinsic lesion, causing the patient's symptoms. A barium enema was then performed, showing many sigmoid bowel diverticula with an area of diverticulitis and spasm in the area of the bladder. The patient responded to conservative medical management. The urinary tract infection was treated with sulfisoxazole, and the patient has remained well on diet and antispasmodics. Biopsy of the bladder lesion showed a chronic cystitis.

2. An inflammatory lesion in the bladder just above the interureteric ridge is often an early manifestation of:
   A. Carcinoma of sigmoid colon
   B. Carcinoma of uterus
   C. Carcinoma of prostate
   D. Carcinoma of ovary

3. An inflammatory lesion in the bladder on its left lateral wall is often an early manifestation of:
   A. Carcinoma of sigmoid colon
   B. Carcinoma of uterus
   C. Carcimoma of prostate
   D. Carcinoma of ovary

4. An inflammatory lesion of the bladder on the trigone is often an early manifestation of:
   A. Carcinoma of sigmoid colon
   B. Carcinoma of uterus
   C. Carcinoma of prostate
   D. Carcinoma of ovary

5. The suspicion of the "herald" lesion should be heightened if:
   A. The vesical lesion is single rather than multiple
   B. It is slightly raised and shaggy
   C. It is somewhat irregular and surrounded by bulbous edema
   D. Telangiectasia is present
   E. All of these

ANSWERS AND DISCUSSION

1. (C) Gross terminal hematuria may be secondary to pathology in the urethra or the bladder. Bladder tumors will not infrequently present with only terminal hematuria and not total hematuria. The fact that the patient has only terminal hematuria does not rule out the possibility of upper tract pathology, especially if the blood in the urine is secondary to a bladder tumor.

2. (B) Melicow and Uson coined the term "herald" lesions of
3. (A) the bladder to indicate certain urothelial and submu-
4. (C) cosal changes in the bladder induced by cancerous or
        inflammatory processes originating outside the bladder

wall. This was found to be particularly true when changes were confined to certain localized areas in the bladder. These were referred to as "critical areas." "Herald" lesions in the posterior wall above the interureteric ridge were most often found to be secondary to disease in the uterus, either corpus or cervix. Of those on the left lateral wall, either sigmoid colon or rectum, and around the bladder neck and trigone, the prostate was most often the offending external organ.

5. (E) All of the listed answers are standard criteria for suspicion of a "herald" lesion. A bulge may also be present and, with advancement of the process, the area may become ulcerated and show signs of necrotic debris. Later, fistula formation may occur, with mucous and fecal material being seen in the bladder. With any of the above findings, investigation must proceed by evaluation of the surrounding structures mentioned, to establish a diagnosis.

REFERENCE

1. Melicow MM and Uson AC: The "herald" lesion of the bladder: A lesion which portends the approach of cancer or inflammation from outside the bladder. J Urol 85:543, Apr., 1961.

CHAPTER V

TUBERCULOSIS

INTRODUCTION

Renal tuberculosis, like tuberculosis in other organs, is a chronic granulomatous infection caused by Mycobacterium tuberculosis. It is a disease of young people, with 60% of the patients in the 20-40-year age group. Pulmonary tuberculosis can be demonstrated in approximately 40% of the cases. Although the disease is usually manifested by unilateral changes, the process is bilateral in the great majority of cases, as demonstrated by Medlar in 1926. The etiology is hematogenous, organisms reaching the kidney via the blood stream through the respiratory or gastrointestinal system. If the bacteria are of sufficient virulence and/or the host resistance is decreased, the organisms lodge in the medulla, and the typical granulomatous process occurs with the eventual destruction of renal tissue. This process generally begins in the tip of the papilla, and the earliest pyelographic findings are those of papillary destruction or scarring of the major calyx. With progression of the process, caseation necrosis occurs, producing large abscess cavities and eventual nonfunction of the kidney. Ulceration into the calyceal system eventually occurs, the renal pelvis ureter becomes involved, and with further progression downwards, the bladder, seminal vesicles, prostate, and epididymis are commonly involved. There is a tendency to healing fibrosis, and with involvement of the ureter this fibrosis can lead to obstruction and hydroureteronephrosis with eventual destruction of the whole kidney. This is sometimes seen with therapy; therefore, it is advised to periodically dilate the involved ureter in patients on therapy. Tuberculous cystitis occurs in 70-80% of renal cases, giving rise to symptoms of frequency, urgency, dysuria, and hematuria.

The diagnosis can best be made by isolation of the tubercle bacilli from the urine. Bladder biopsy and staining of the organism in the typical granulomatous lesion can also lead to diagnosis.

The treatment of renal tuberculosis is primarily medical, and requires 18-24 months of triple therapy. Success of treatment can be expected in 95% of early cases after the above regimen and a second course of therapy is recommended for those who relapse. Rarely is surgery indicated.

CASE 27: 32-YEAR-OLD MALE WITH FREQUENCY, URGENCY AND DYSURIA

HISTORY

A 32-year-old male was seen because of frequency, urgency, and dysuria of several months duration. He denied any history of fever, hematuria, or flank pain. There was no history of exposure to tuberculosis. He had lived in the Middle East most of his life.

PHYSICAL EXAMINATION

The blood pressure was 140/70. Heart and chest were normal. There was no costovertebral angle tenderness. Abdomen was normal. The genitalia and prostate were normal.

LABORATORY DATA

Urinalysis revealed 6-8 WBCs per high power field, and no red cells were seen. There was 1+ albumin and no casts. Routine urine culture showed no growth on three occasions. Blood urea nitrogen was normal. An intravenous urogram showed normal upper tracts bilaterally. In the right lower ureter there was an area of stricture formation. Cystoscopy revealed diffuse areas of hemorrhagic cystitis; a right retrograde ureteropyelogram confirmed the presence of the ureteral stricture (Fig. 27.1). A bladder biopsy showed only nonspecific inflammatory reaction.

CLINICAL COURSE

Four urine specimens were collected for culture for Mycobacterium tuberculosis. Two were positive. He was started on triple therapy and has remained asymptomatic since. He will remain on therapy for two years.

QUESTIONS

1. Pyuria and a negative urine culture is:
    A. Always indicative of tuberculosis
    B. Sometimes indicative of tuberculosis
    C. Usually indicates infection
    D. Should be repeated since the patient probably took antibiotics

2. The earliest pyelographic evidence of tuberculosis is:
    A. Ureteral stricture with obstruction

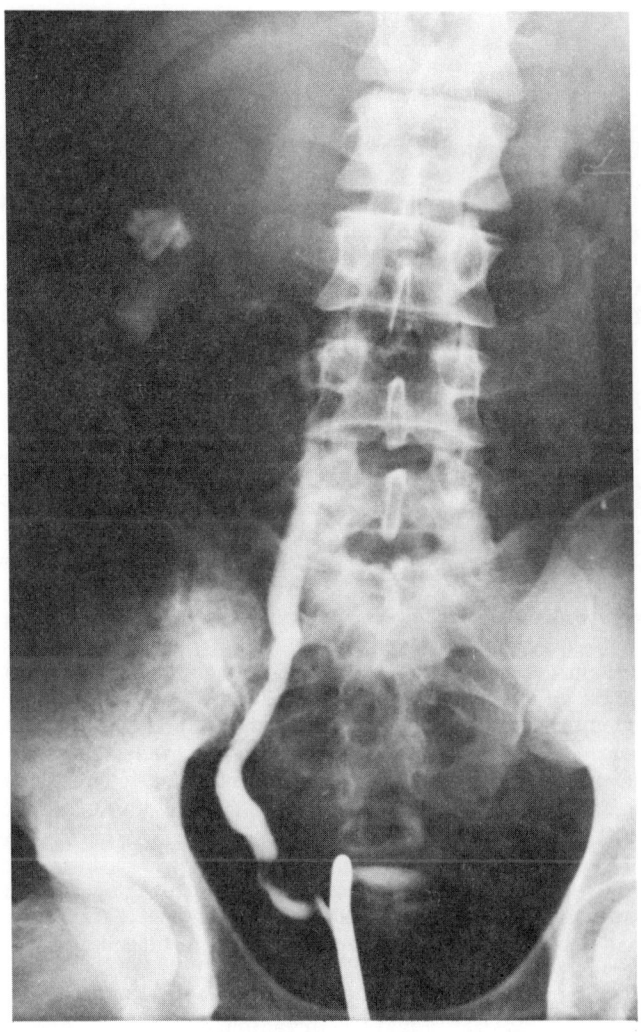

FIG. 27.1: Right retrograde pyelogram showing stricture of ureter secondary to tuberculosis.

136/ Case 27 — Tuberculosis

    B. Calcification in the renal parenchyma
    C. Papillary destruction, irregularity of the minor calyx
    D. Infundibular scarring

3. The etiology of renal tuberculosis is:
    A. Hematogenous
    B. By direct extension
    C. By lymphatic spread
    D. In retrograde fashion following bladder infection

4. Bladder irritative symptoms:
    A. Rarely occur with tuberculosis
    B. Are quite commonly associated with renal tuberculosis
    C. Almost never are associated with renal tuberculosis
    D. Indicate a grave prognosis if associated with renal tuberculosis

5. With minimal involvement of the kidney and the presence of a positive urine culture for mycobacterium tuberculosis, the preferred method of management would be:
    A. Streptomycin, INH and PAS
    B. Two drugs are as good as three
    C. Ethambutol, INH and cycloserine
    D. INH for two years

ANSWERS AND DISCUSSION

1. (B) In the male especially, the presence of pyuria and a negative urine culture should lead one to the suspicion of the possibility of a prostatitis; this should be ruled out by examination of the prostate as well as a two glass test for the possibility of pyuria only in the first glass. This would indicate infection below the level of the bladder neck and probable prostatitis.

    In the absence of this, however, with pyuria and no growth on urine culture, tuberculosis must be a primary suspect and ruled out by numerous cultures for the offending organism.

2. (C) As described in the introduction, tuberculosis is generally blood-borne and the organism lodges in the medulla of the kidney involving first the area of the papilla, causing accumulation of contrast material in this area with blunting of the calyx.

3. (A)

Tuberculosis

4. (B) Bladder irritative symptoms can occur in 70-80% of the patients with renal tuberculosis and are often the presenting symptoms, as in the case cited here. This rarely, if ever, affects the overall prognosis.

5. (C) Triple therapy is indicated in all cases of renal tuberculosis and oral medication should be given in one dose (usually in the morning). Pyridoxine should always be added to the regimen when INH is included. Streptomycin is rarely indicated today because of its severe side-effects.

CASE 28: 29-YEAR-OLD FEMALE WITH DIFFICULTY IN VOIDING

HISTORY

This is a 29-year-old black female with a 2-year history of difficulty in voiding, frequency every 2 hours, and nocturia five times with marked dysuria and left flank pain. She denied hematuria. No fever. Past medical history: appendectomy and T&A. Otherwise, negative.

PHYSICAL EXAMINATION

Blood pressure 170/120. Mild-left CVA tenderness, otherwise negative.

LABORATORY DATA

IVP showed marked hydronephrosis on the left with dilation of the ureter to the juxtavesicular area. There was mild dilation on the right (Fig. 28.1). Cystoscopy revealed diffuse hemorrhagic cystitis. Bladder capacity was only 70cc. Urine showed many WBCs; routine culture showed no growth. Two out of three urine cultures for AFB showed Mycobacterium tuberculosis. She was placed on triple therapy.

QUESTIONS

1. The plan at this time should be:
    A. Continue triple therapy for 2 years and repeat the study (culture and IVP)
    B. Continue therapy for one year and repeat the studies
    C. Continue therapy for four months and repeat the studies
    D. If the patient's symptoms improve she can be watched safely for one year before repeat radiographic studies are done

2. Triple therapy in renal tuberculosis:
    A. Almost always results in complete arrest of the infection
    B. Can be associated with scarring in critical areas and cause obstruction
    C. Is associated with few side-effects
    D. Usually has only minimal effect on lower tract symptoms

3. Obstructive uropathy associated with ureteral scarring should be treated by:
    A. Ureteral dilation at periodic intervals

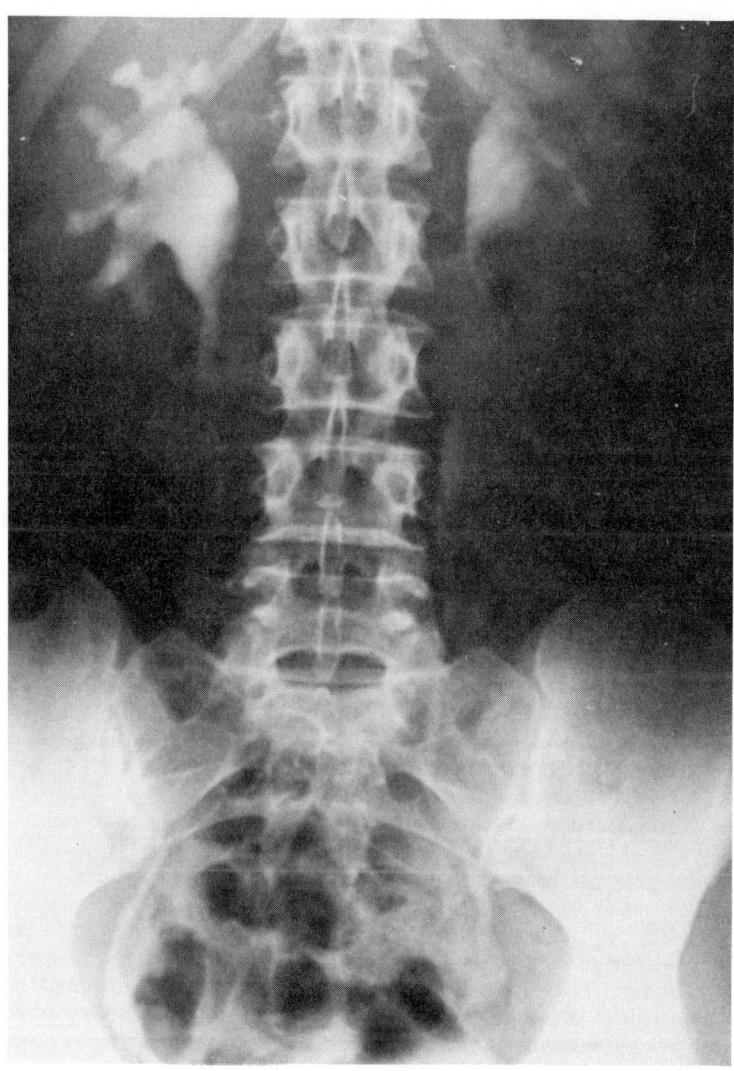

FIG. 28.1: Intravenous urogram before therapy was begun.

B. Continue therapy for one year and repeat the studies
C. Continue therapy for four months and repeat the studies
D. If the patient's symptoms improve, she can be watched safely for one year before repeat radiographic studies are done

CLINICAL COURSE

Her voiding pattern changed gradually within 2 months. She developed a bladder capacity of 240cc and would go several hours without voiding. An intravenous urogram was repeated after 4 months of therapy; the dilation on the left side was markedly increased (Fig. 28.2). The ureter was dilated to 7F, with obstruction met 4cm proximal to the left ureteral orifice. Dilations were carried out at 4-month intervals and urograms repeated. She remained on antituberculous therapy for 2 years. Repeat cultures at 4-month intervals were negative for AFB. Urogram two years after completing therapy (Fig. 28.3) is shown. She remained asymptomatic and has had a normal voiding pattern for the past ten years.

4. Which of the following are indicative of urinary tract tuberculosis?
   A. Ureteral obstruction with pyuria
   B. Painless epididymitis
   C. Severe symptoms of cystitis and negative cultures
   D. All of the above

5. Nephrectomy for renal tuberculosis is indicated:
   A. In severe cases with a good contralateral kidney
   B. For a nonfunctioning kidney
   C. To cure the patient completely
   D. Rarely, if ever indicated

ANSWERS AND DISCUSSION

1. (C) As illustrated beautifully in this case, things can get worse after starting therapy in renal and ureteral tuberculosis. Repeat excretory urogram should be performed four months after initiating therapy and probably every four months during therapy. Some recommend routine ureteral dilation even in the absence of demonstrable obstruction.

2. (B) As illustrated in this case, scarring and obstruction do occur. There are always side-effects in any medications given and these must always be borne in mind and looked for. As here, lower urinary tract symptoms are generally

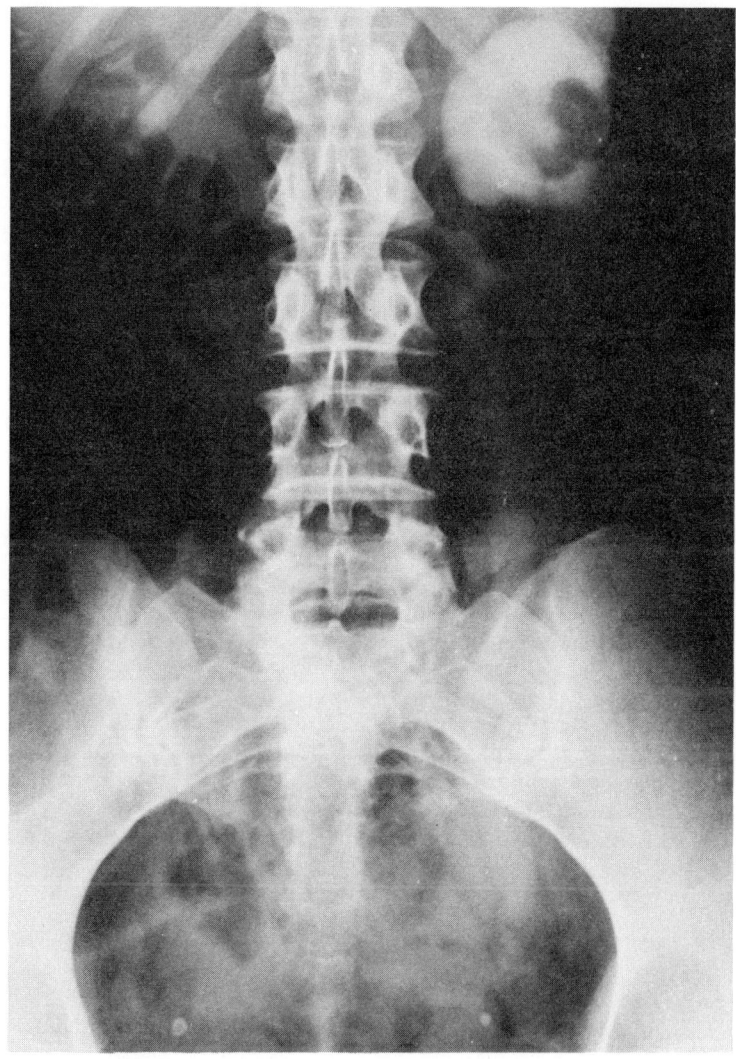

FIG. 28.2: Intravenous urogram after four months of therapy showing increased dilatation of the left ureter and hydroureteronephrosis.

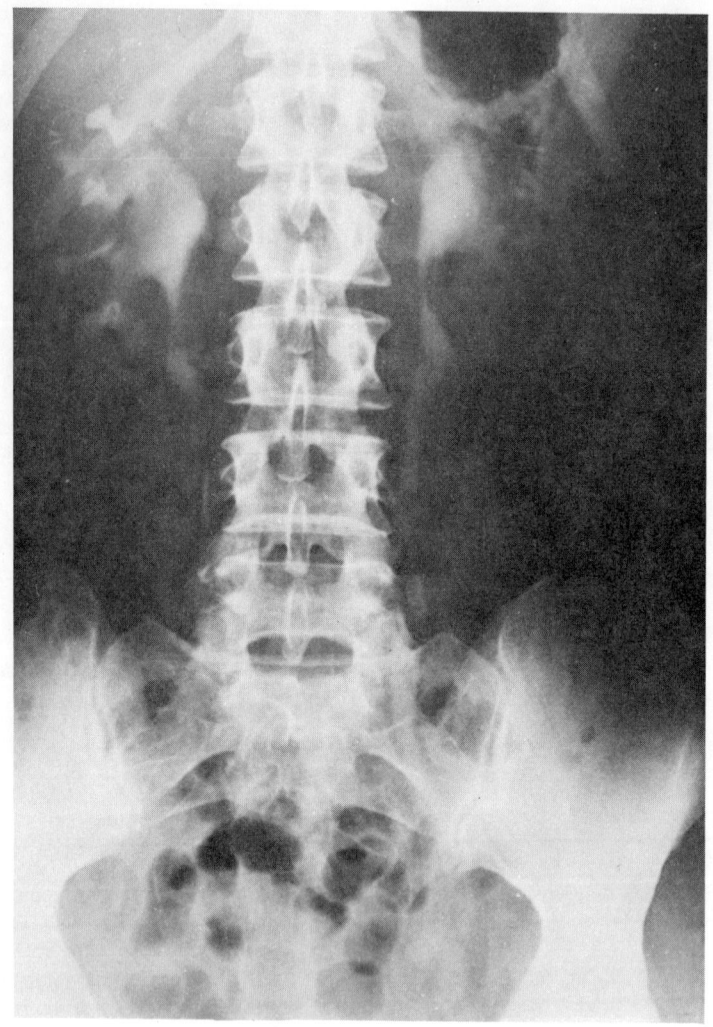

FIG. 28.3: Intravenous urogram after two years of triple antituberculous therapy and ureteral dilations at 4-month intervals.

markedly improved after therapy is instituted.

3. (A) As illustrated in this case, good results can be obtained and usually are with periodic ureteral dilations. Occasionally, this cannot be accomplished and reimplantation is required if the obstruction is in the lower ureter. If the stricture is very short, ureteroureterostomy could be performed, but this would be hazardous in a severely diseased ureter. Transureteroureterostomy would not be recommended if there was no evidence of disease in the opposite kidney or ureter.

4. (D) All of the conditions stated should bring tuberculosis into the differential diagnosis, and this should be ruled out by multiple serial cultures.

5. (D) Nephrectomy is rarely, if ever indicated in renal tuberculosis. Occasionally, perinephric abscess, requiring nephrectomy, may occur; but in the multiple antibiotic era this would be a most unusual occurrence. If the kidney has no function whatsoever and is accompanied by renal pain, nephrectomy may then be necessary.

CASE 29: 45-YEAR-OLD MALE WITH PYURIA

HISTORY

A 45-year-old male was first seen in June, 1959, because his family physician found pyuria on a routine urinalysis. He stated that in 1943 he fractured his right shoulder while prisoner in a concentration camp. In 1948, he developed a cutaneous fistula from this same shoulder, which was diagnosed as tuberculosis and treated with chemotherapy.

In 1954, he developed bilateral swellings of the testicles and terminal hematuria. He apparently was not treated for tuberculosis at this time. When he was originally seen by us in 1959, he complained of frequency, urgency, and dysuria.

PHYSICAL EXAMINATION

There was a healed, cutaneous fistula of the right shoulder. The chest was clear to percussion and auscultation. There was bilateral induration of the epididymis with no tenderness. The testicles and prostate were normal.

LABORATORY DATA

The urine had 10-12 WBCs per high power field. BUN was 22 mg%. A routine urine culture showed no growth. Intravenous urogram revealed severe pyelonephritic changes on the left, probably secondary to tuberculosis (Fig. 29.1). Six cultures for tuberculosis were taken and all were positive.

CLINICAL COURSE

The patient was given INH, PAS, and streptomycin, as well as pyridoxine for a period of two years.

His urine cultures have remained sterile for tuberculosis, but the severe pyelonephritic changes in the left kidney are unchanged.

DISCUSSION

This case represents one of far-advanced tuberculosis with both bone and renal disease as well as healed pulmonary disease. The induration in the epididymis probably represents tuberculosis infection, even though this was not apparently recognized when it first appeared in 1954.

Multiple positive cultures have been shown to carry a poorer prognosis for recurrence of disease, but in this man with very severe disease, he has apparently not had a recurrence in ten years after one course of triple therapy.

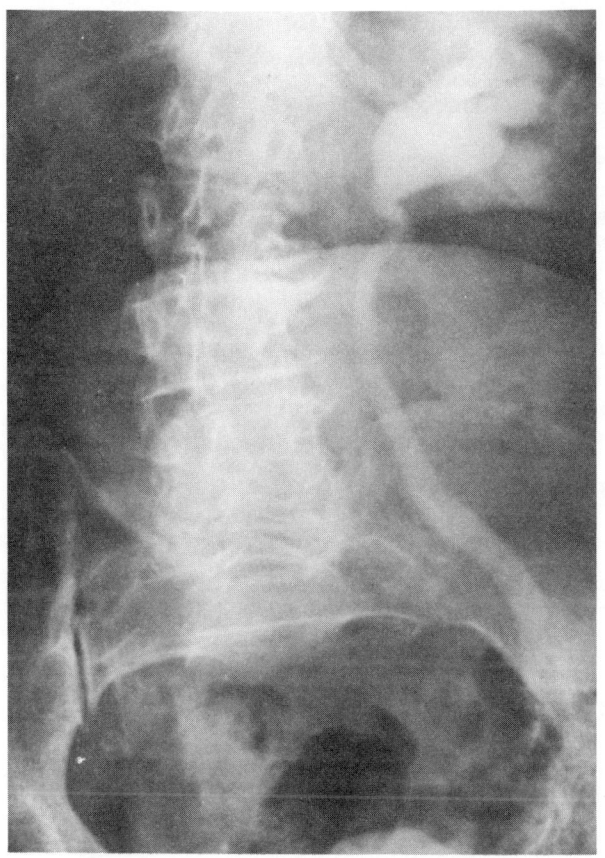

FIG. 29.1: Intravenous urogram.

REFERENCE

1. Lattimer JK, and Wechsler M: Genitourinary tuberculosis, Chapter 15. In: Campbell's Urology, Harrison JH, et al. (eds.), W. B. Saunders Company, Philadelphia, 1978, p. 557.

CHAPTER VI

RENAL TUMORS

INTRODUCTION

Benign tumors of the kidney are very common, but rarely become manifest during life, being commonly found at autopsy. The most common type is adenoma. Fibroma, lipoma, myoma and angioma, or combinations thereof, are other types of benign renal tumors (Case 33 illustrates this type). Occasionally, even minute angiomata of the renal pelvis may be the cause of troublesome bleeding, making diagnosis extremely difficult.

Cysts of the kidney are generally classified as follows:

1. Congenital polycystic disease
    a) Infantile form
    b) Adult form
2. Multicystic kidney
3. Simple serous (solitary cyst)
4. Pyelogenic cyst
5. Peripelvic cyst

In a discussion of renal tumors, the above are clinically important only from the standpoint of differentiation of cyst from tumor. With the newer diagnostic modalities, this differentiation can be accurately made with a high degree of dependability.

Malignant tumors of the kidney are relatively uncommon, and comprise 3% of all malignancies of the body. Ninety percent occur past the age of forty. The three major varieties are adenocarcinoma of the renal parenchyma (85%), (commonly miscalled "hypernephroma"); transitional cell carcinoma of the pelvis and calyceal system (8-10%), and nephroblastoma, or Wilms' tumor (5-6%). The remainder are sarcomatous tumors.

Adenocarcinoma, or more commonly, clear cell carcinoma, arises in the cortex of the kidney, and compresses the renal parenchyma around it, forming a false capsule. It is characteristically grossly golden yellow in color (due to large, lipid-containing cells). Calcification can sometimes be present. Histologically, there are sheets of large, clear cells, each with a small, darkly stained nucleus. The cells resemble adrenal cortical cells, accounting for the misnomer of "hypernephroma."

With continued, untreated growth of the tumor, local invasion spreads to involve the branches of the renal vein, then spreads to the main renal vein and into the vena cava. Tumors have been reported extending into the right atrium. Metastases, in order of frequency, are to the lungs, lymph nodes, bone, liver, and brain.

Transitional cell carcinomas arise in the pelvic and calyceal epithelial lining, and are similar in etiology and morphology to transitional cell tumors of the ureter and bladder. In contrast to bladder tumors, however, most of those of the kidney and pelvis are malignant, and have early invasion with metastasis.

Wilms' tumor, or nephroblastoma, is a renal malignancy of childhood found, ordinarily, in children under the age of six. It is a rare tumor; but it comprises one-third of the malignant tumors of infants, and 15% of all tumors under the age of 15. These generally present as a large abdominal mass, sometimes occupying most of the abdominal cavity, with compression of the remainder of the abdominal contents.

The classical triad of renal tumor (hematuria, abdominal mass, and pain) are rarely seen together. They are generally very late symptoms. Hematuria, the presenting symptom in more than half the cases, is generally intermittent, and should be investigated as soon as it is manifest. The onset follows invasion of the calyceal system by the tumor. It is most common in transitional cell tumors of the pelvis, and rarely occurs in nephroblastoma. Flank mass is most common in nephroblastoma, and rarely occurs with transitional cell carcinoma of the pelvis, but may be seen fairly commonly with adenocarcinoma. The presence of tumor may first become manifest by a pulmonary or osseous metastasis. Other unusual manifestations are unexplained fever, anemia, or, paradoxically, polycythemia (3% of cases of renal carcinoma), or wasting.

Investigations of patients with the above symptoms should generally progress along the following lines. Excretory urography will demonstrate the presence and general function of the kidneys. Tumors of the renal parenchyma would be evident by separation, elongation, or flattening of the calyces. Filling defects within the pelvis may be indicative of transitional cell carcinoma,

Renal Tumors

but would have to be differentiated from radiolucent calculus or blood clot following bleeding.

The next step would be cystoscopy and retrograde ureteropyelography, if intravenous urography fails to define the morphology of the collecting system adequately. This will rule out the possible other causes of hematuria from the lower urinary tract and, if performed at the time of bleeding, may localize the bleeding to one or the other kidney.

Following the above, nephrotomography may be performed. This procedure can be very helpful in differentiating cyst from tumor, or for such conditions as renal hilar lipomatosis where tumor may be suspect. If this diagnosis can be made on tomography, no further treatment would be necessary. Radioisotope scanning of the kidneys is another valuable adjunctive tool.

The addition of sonography and computerized axial tomography has added significantly to the urologist's differential diagnosis of cyst from tumor. If a cyst is apparent on this study, a cyst puncture can be performed, with analysis of the fluid for evidence of malignancy by cytology, as well as enzyme studies (see Case 36).

Invaluable to the urologist, in treating renal tumors, are aortography and renal angiography. Not only will this differentiate benign cyst from tumor in a high percentage of cases, but it is of extreme importance in planning the approach to be used for radical nephrectomy for malignant disease. In this procedure, all perinephric fat and fascia are removed, along with the lymph nodes of the hilar region, as well as those around the vena cava in the case of right renal tumors, and the aorta in left tumors.

Renal Tumors

CASE 30: 69-YEAR-OLD MALE WITH HEMATURIA

HISTORY

A 69-year-old white male was admitted with his first episode of gross total painless hematuria. He denied difficulty in voiding, thin stream, or frequency. There was no history of weakness, poor appetite, or weight loss. On questioning, he related a history of dull right flank pain of several months duration. Past history and review of systems were negative.

PHYSICAL EXAMINATION

Blood pressure was 140/80. The abdomen was soft, and there was a nontender, hard, smooth mass palpable in the right upper quadrant of the abdomen that moved with respiration. There was no costovertebral angle tenderness. The remainder of the physical examination was negative.

QUESTIONS

1. Which of the following are considered to be the classical triad of renal carcinoma?
    A. Hematuria, flank mass, and weight loss
    B. Hematuria, polycythemia, and fever
    C. Hematuria, flank pain, and a mass
    D. Anemia, hematuria, and flank mass
    E. The classical triad almost never exists

2. The differential diagnosis in this patient should include:
    A. Renal cell carcinoma
    B. Angiomyolipoma
    C. Transitional cell carcinoma
    D. A & C
    E. All of the above

3. Clinical findings associated with renal cell carcinoma can include:
    A. Fever
    B. Hypercalcemia
    C. Polycythemia
    D. Amyloidosis
    E. All of the above

LABORATORY DATA

Hematocrit 46%. Urinalysis showed 10-12 RBC/HPF and 1 + albumin. Blood urea nitrogen 14mg%. Creatinine 0.9%. Urine culture: no growth. Chest x-ray, metastatic bone survey and liver scan showed no evidence of metastases. An intravenous urogram with tomography revealed a right renal mass. Selective angiogram (Fig. 30.1) showed typical abnormal vasculature of neoplasm. Cystoscopy showed a normal bladder. Inferior vena cavagram was normal.

CLINICAL COURSE

A radical right nephrectomy was performed through a Nagamatsu incision. The patient has done well since that time, and there is no evidence of metastatic disease six years postsurgery.

4. In a nephrectomy for renal cell carcinoma, which should be accomplished first?
   A. Ligation of renal vein
   B. Ligation of renal artery
   C. Both of the above together
   D. Ligation of the ureter

5. To be considered cured, survival from renal cell carcinoma should be at least:
   A. Three years
   B. Five years
   C. Ten years
   D. Twenty years

6. Abnormal liver chemistries (elevated SGOT, SGPT, bilirubin, and alkaline phosphatase), when found preoperatively in renal cell carcinoma, indicate:
   A. A poor prognosis
   B. A liver biopsy should be done
   C. Concomitant hepatic disease is present
   D. Is of no prognostic value

7. All of the following should be removed at the time of radical nephrectomy, except:
   A. Gerota's fat and fascia
   B. Ipsilateral adrenal gland
   C. Lymph nodes from the crus of the diaphragm to the bifurcation of the aorta
   D. The entire ureter

8. The 5-year survival rate for renal cell carcinoma is:
   A. 15-25%
   B. 25-35%
   C. 35-45%

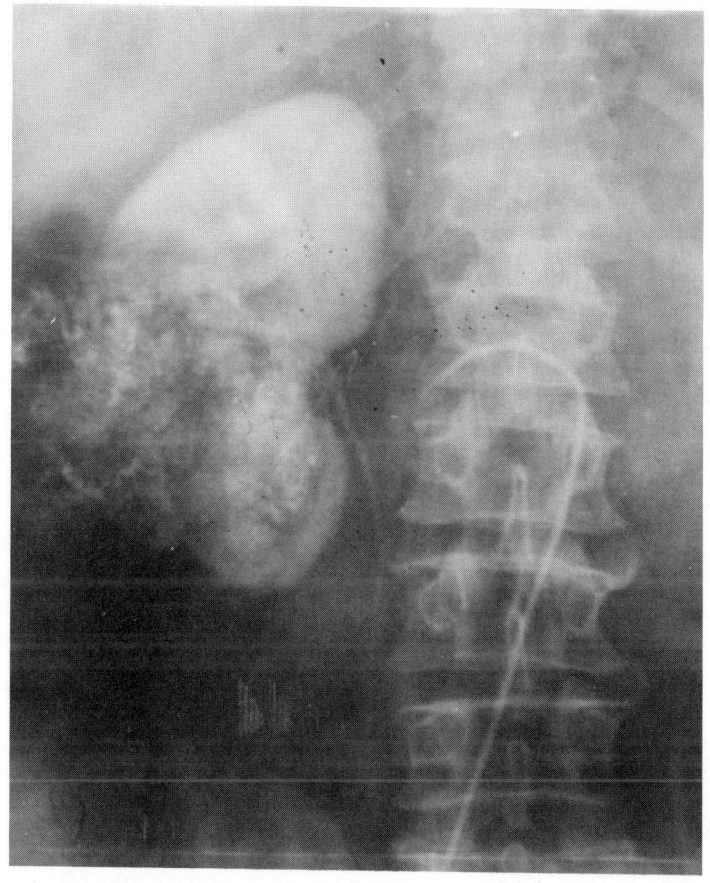

FIG. 30.1: Right renal angiogram demonstrating mass at lower pole of kidney.

D. 55-65%
E. 75-80%

9. The choice of chemotherapy for renal cell carcinoma would be:
   A. 5-Fluorouracil
   B. Actinomycin D
   C. Vincristine
   D. A combination of the above
   E. Medroxyprogresterone or testosterone

10. Involvement of the renal vein in renal cell carcinoma indicates:
    A. A poor prognosis
    B. Inoperability
    C. Has no prognostic significance
    D. Should not deter surgery

ANSWERS AND DISCUSSION

1. (C) The classical triad of renal cell carcinoma is hematuria, flank pain, and a palpable mass. These are rarely seen in one individual, such as in this case, and, when seen, the tumor is generally in an advanced stage. Anemia is commonly associated with renal cell tumors, and, this too, is generally indicative of an advanced stage of the disease. Polycythemia, although much discussed, occurs only 2-4% of the time. Fever is commonly associated with this neoplasm, and is often the presenting symptom. Weight loss would also be a very late symptom.

2. (E) The three lesions mentioned should all be considered in the differential diagnosis, as they can all have the history, as well as physical findings described.

3. (E) In a series of over 1,000 cases at the Mayo Clinic, 11% of patients with renal cell carcinoma had fever as a presenting symptom. Hypercalcemia can occur with renal cell tumor and, at times, symptoms referable to this (i.e., weakness, lethargy, polyuria, constipation, etc.), may be the presenting complaint. The mechanism involved is postulated to be secretion of a parathormone-like substance by the tumor, but this has not been definitely proven. Polycythemia, as mentioned above, occurs in 2-4% of cases. The mechanism believed to be responsible for this is believed to be humeral via an erythropoietic stimulating hormone by the tumor. Secondary amyloidosis is very rare with renal cell carcinoma, but has been reported to occur.

4. (B) The renal artery should be clamped first. By doing so, one precludes the trapping of blood in the tumor. This also alters the hemodynamics somewhat, and makes the possibility of tumor emboli less likely. Of course, the tumor should be manipulated as little as possible.

5. (C) Renal cell carcinoma is an unusual tumor, in that patients can live for a comparatively long period of time being apparently free of tumor, only to die after five or more years of metastatic disease. It is for this reason that Robson recommends a 10-15 year follow-up to properly assess results.

6. (D) Evidence of hepatic dysfunction by the biochemical tests noted is now a well known occurrence. Generally, these will return to normal after nephrectomy, and do not alter the prognosis of the cancer.

7. (D) Radical nephrectomy includes the kidney and surrounding fat and fascia, including the ipsilateral adrenal gland and lymph nodes surrounding the vena cava and aorta from the crus of the diaphragm down to the bifurcation of the aorta. The ureter is generally divided as it crosses the common iliac artery.

8. (C) The five-year survival rates reported generally range from 35-45%, the highest reported by Robson.

9. (E) Chemotherapy is of little value in clear cell carcinoma. There have been reports of suppression of tumor growth with medroxyprogesterone.

10. (D) Involvement of the renal vein certainly makes the operation more difficult, but should not deter the surgeon from attempting to cure the patient. This is generally accomplished by isolating the vena cava above and below the affected renal vein, as well as the opposite renal vein, and opening the vena cava to remove the tumor clot en bloc with the tumor. Naturally, the prognosis becomes much graver.

REFERENCES

1. Scott R (ed.): Current Controversies in Urologic Management, Chapter 2, W.B. Saunders Company, Philadelphia, 1972.

2. Freed SZ and Gliedman ML: The removal of renal carcinoma thrombosis extending into the right atrium. J Urol 113:163, 1975.

3. Bloom HJG: Medroxyprogesterone acetate (Provera) in the treatment of metastatic renal carcinoma. Br J Cancer 25: 250, 1971.

4. Robson CI, Churchill BM, and Anderson W: The results of radical nephrectomy for renal cell carcinoma. J Urol 101: 297-301, 1969.

Renal Tumors

CASE 31: 54-YEAR-OLD FEMALE WITH FLANK PAIN AND HEMATURIA

HISTORY

A 54-year-old female presented with a 2-month history of left flank pain and hematuria. There were no other urinary symptoms. She had a left pneumonectomy 10 years prior to admission for bronchiectasis, with no recurrent symptoms or pulmonary disability. She had had a 15-pound weight loss over the previous several months.

PHYSICAL EXAMINATION

Unremarkable, except for an old thoracoplasty with the heart shifted to the left.

LABORATORY DATA

Hematocrit 38%. CBC normal. Blood urea nitrogen 10mg%. Electrolytes normal. Urinalysis revealed many RBCs and WBCs/HPF. Albumin 2+. Urine culture showed no growth. Chest x-ray showed no evidence of disease in the remaining right lung. Metastatic survey was negative. Pulmonary function studies showed good compensation with adequate reserve. An intravenous urogram showed a normal right kidney (Fig. 31.1). The left upper collecting system was compressed, and filled with an irregular mass. Cystoscopy showed no evidence of bladder tumor, and a retrograde ureteropyelogram revealed no evidence of tumor in the ureter (Fig. 31.2). A left renal angiogram showed some, but minimal, tumor vasculature between the left middle and upper poles (Fig. 31.3). Renal venogram was normal (Fig. 31.4).

CRITICAL COURSE

The patient underwent transperitoneal nephroureterectomy. Pathologic report was infiltrating transitional cell carcinoma. There was no evidence of metastases at the time of surgery.

QUESTIONS

1. Which of the following is the most helpful in pre-op diagnosis of a transitional cell Ca of renal pelvis?
   A. Urine cytology from affected kidney
   B. Renal angiogram
   C. Infusion intravenous urogram
   D. Nephrotomography

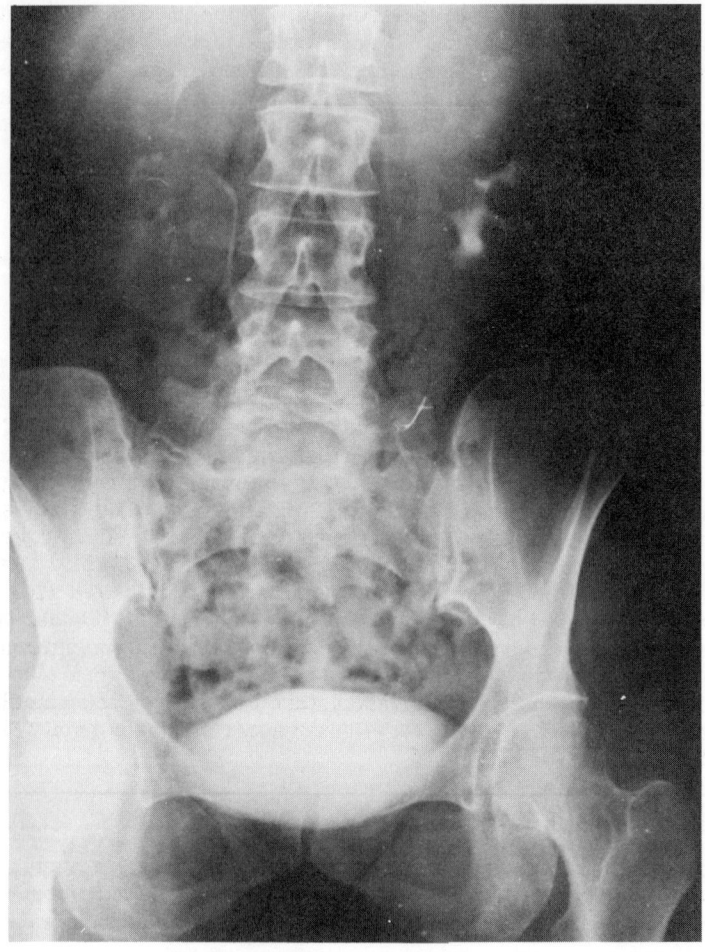

FIG. 31.1: Intravenous urogram showing depression of the left collecting system and filling defect in the pelvis.

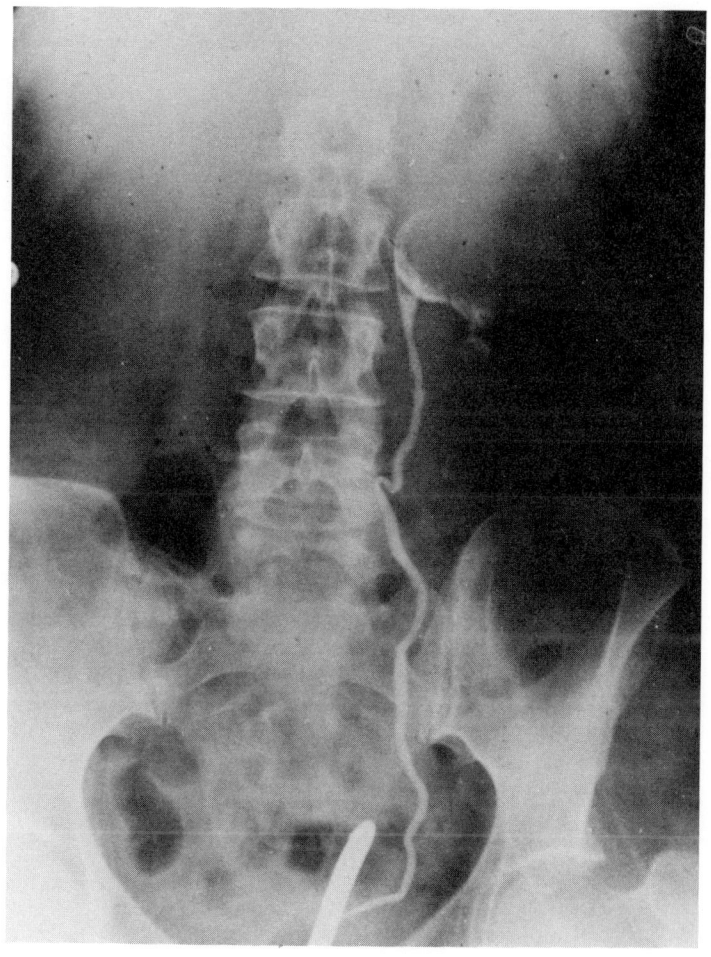

FIG. 31.2: Left retrograde pyelogram. There is a marked filling defect in the renal pelvis. There is no evidence of tumor in the ureter.

158/ Case 31 Renal Tumors

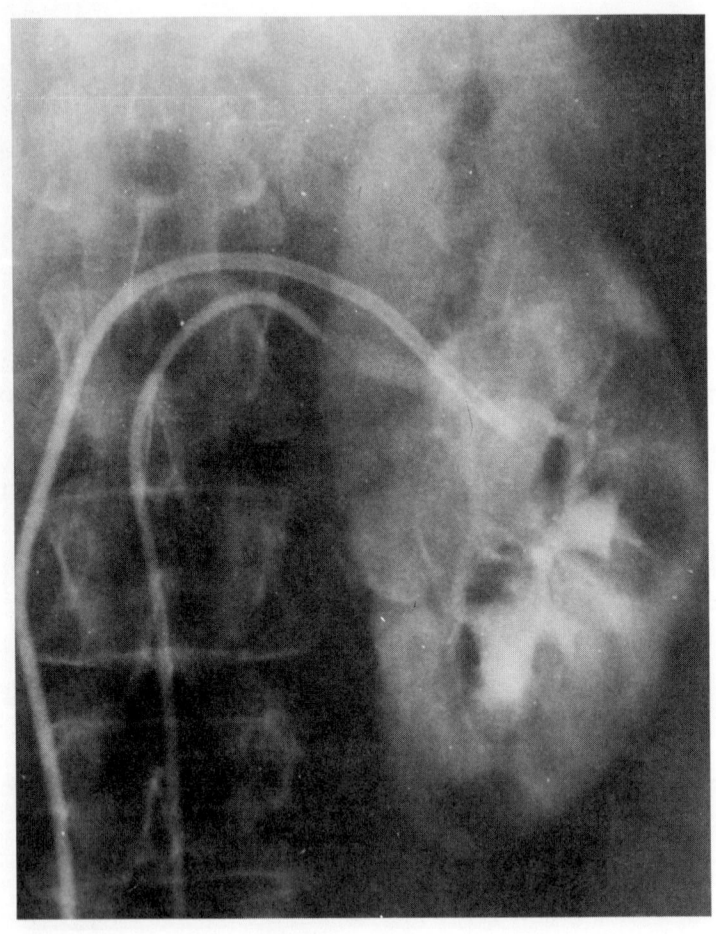

FIG. 31.3: There is a catheter in the renal artery (lower) and renal vein. Arterial injection shows only minimal vascularization of the tumor.

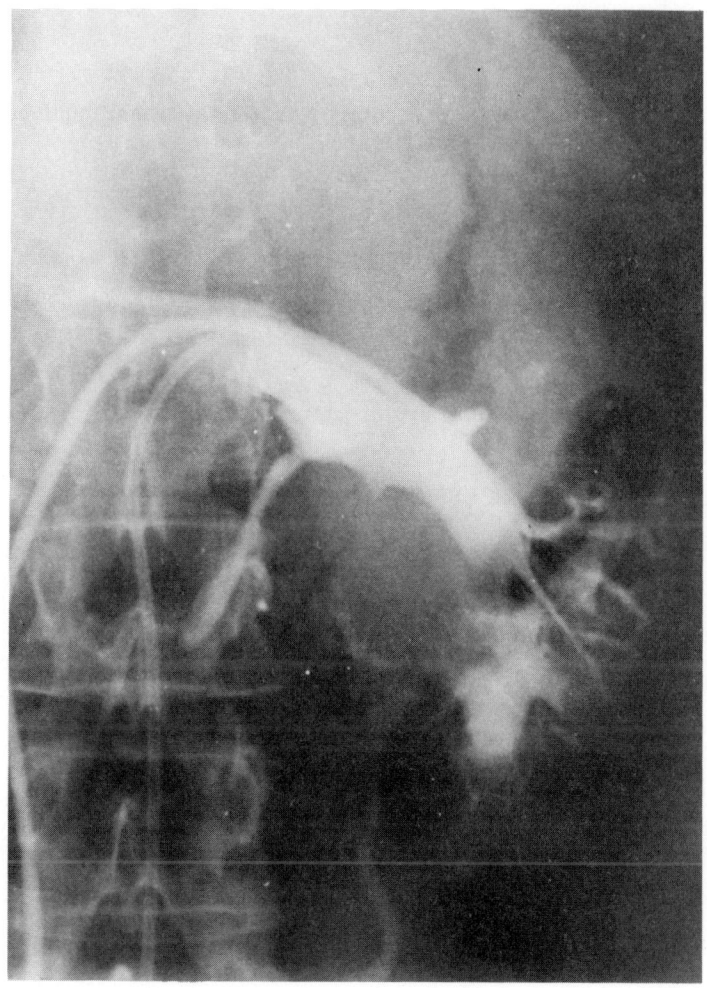

FIG. 31.4: Renal venogram shows no evidence of invasion of left vein by tumor.

2. The proper therapy for transitional cell carcinoma of the pelvis is:
   A. Excision and end-to-end anastomosis
   B. Nephroureterectomy
   C. Radiotherapy
   D. A & B

3. The most common presenting symptom of transitional cell tumor of the renal pelvis is:
   A. Pain in flank
   B. Flank mass
   C. Hematuria
   D. Associated with bladder tumor

4. The most important consideration in prediction of prognosis in transitional cell carcinoma of the renal pelvis is:
   A. Grade of tumor
   B. Stage of tumor
   C. Whether a total ureterectomy was done
   D. A & B

ANSWERS AND DISCUSSION

1. (C) An infusion intravenous urogram should show good filling of the entire collecting system, with the typical filling defect seen in the renal pelvis for transitional cell carcinoma. Urine cytology would be helpful, but would not give the exact location of the neoplasm. Angiography and nephrotomography are not as helpful in this type of tumor as they are in tumors of the renal parenchyma.

2. (B) Nephroureterectomy remains the acceptable treatment for transitional cell carcinoma of the renal pelvis. In unusual circumstances, such as tumor in a solitary kidney, or bilateral tumors that are not invasive, local excision may be acceptable.

3. (C) Hematuria is the most common presenting symptom of tumors of the renal pelvis.

4. (D) The grade and stage of the tumor are both of important prognostic significance.

REFERENCE

1. Batata M and Grabstald H: Upper urinary tract urothelial tumors. Urol Clinics of N Amer 3:79, Feb. 1976.

CASE 32: 61-YEAR-OLD MALE WITH HEMATURIA

HISTORY

A 61-year-old male presented with a 2-day history of gross total painless hematuria. There were no other urinary symptoms. His only significant past history was that he had had bilateral inguinal hernias repaired many years ago.

PHYSICAL EXAMINATION

Blood pressure 130/70. Heart and lungs normal. Abdomen normal. There were no organs or masses palpable. Rectal examination showed a mildly enlarged, benign prostate.

LABORATORY DATA

Urinalysis: many RBCs, no WBCs seen. Urine culture, no growth. BUN, creatinine normal. An intravenous urogram revealed a filling defect in the distal right ureter; the upper tracts were otherwise normal (Fig. 32.1). Urine cytology, no evidence of malignant cells.

QUESTIONS

1. The differential diagnosis at this point would include:
   A. Right ureteral calculus
   B. Blood clot in ureter
   C. Ureteral tumor
   D. All of the above

2. The next step in management of this patient should be:
   A. Immediate exploration of ureter
   B. Retrograde ureteropyelogram
   C. Angiography
   D. CT scan

3. A negative urine cytology in this patient:
   A. Rules out neoplasm of urinary tract
   B. Makes neoplasm of urinary tract unlikely
   C. Is probably in error
   D. Is of no value in the differential diagnosis in this case

CLINICAL COURSE

The patient was admitted to the hospital, and a right ureteropyelogram confirmed the presence of the filling defect in the distal

162 / Case 32 Renal Tumors

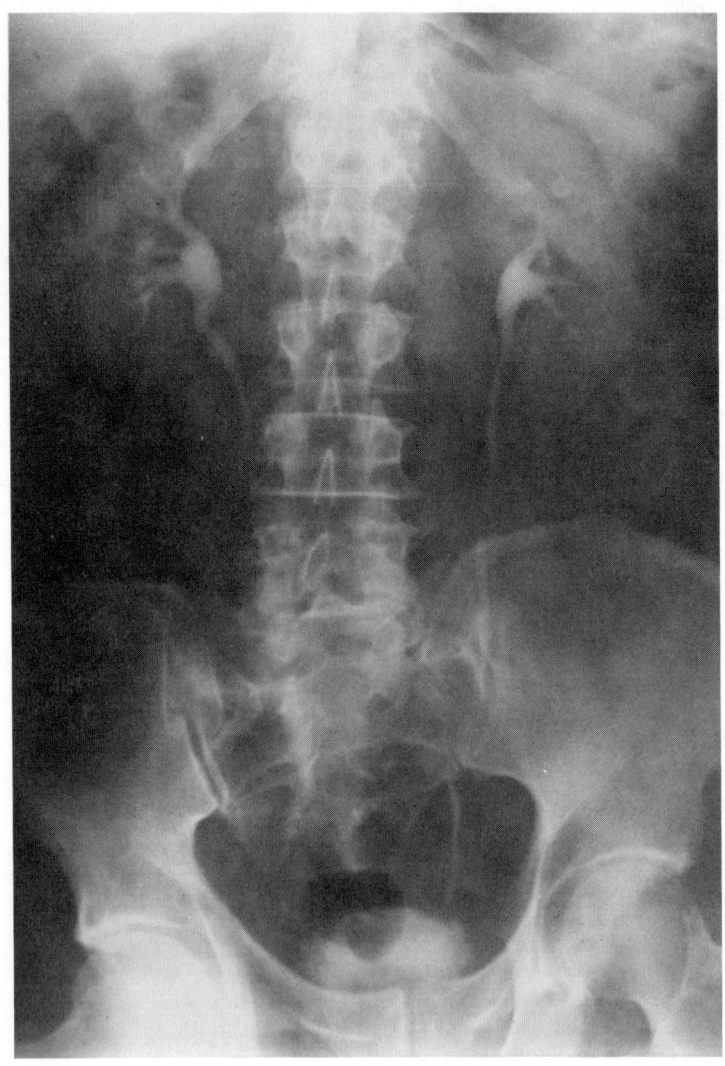

FIG. 32.1: Intravenous urogram showing filling defect in lower ureter, right.

ureter (Fig. 32.2). Exploration of the lower ureter was carried out, a tumor was found, and a right nephroureterectomy was carried out. The patient made an uneventful recovery. He had cystoscopy at 3-month intervals for two years, and at 6-month intervals for two years, without evidence of recurrence. Pathology report was Grade II transitional cell carcinoma of the ureter.

4. The treatment of choice for malignant neoplasm of the distal ureter is:
   A. Excision of the tumor with at least 2cm of normal ureter on either side and end-to-end ureteroureterostomy
   B. Nephroureterectomy
   C. Excision and reimplantation into bladder
   D. Nephroureterectomy with a cuff of bladder

5. The overall 5-year survival rate for primary tumors of the ureter is:
   A. Less than 10%
   B. 10-25%
   C. 25-35%
   D. 35-45%
   E. Over 50%

ANSWERS AND DISCUSSION

1. (D) The differential diagnosis should include all of the possibilities mentioned. An irregular filling defect in the ureter may represent a papillary tumor or an irregular stone.

   A meniscus sign seen at the inferior end of the defect is said to be indicative of a tumor rather than a stone, but this too is not an infallible sign. A ureteral catheter passed retrograde may turn in a downward direction. This has been reported to be indicative of neoplasm as well.

2. (B) As was done here, a retrograde ureteropyelogram should be performed to better delineate the filling defect. Urine can also be collected for cytology directly from the ureter involved. A urine culture can be taken at the same time. Passage of a ureteral catheter, with evidence of "grating" against a hard object, may indicate a calculus. Bleeding seen coming from the suspected orifice would be a very important observation as well.

3. (D) The finding of a negative cytology on one or two specimens by no means rules out the presence of a tumor. This is especially so in the presence of lower grade tumors where

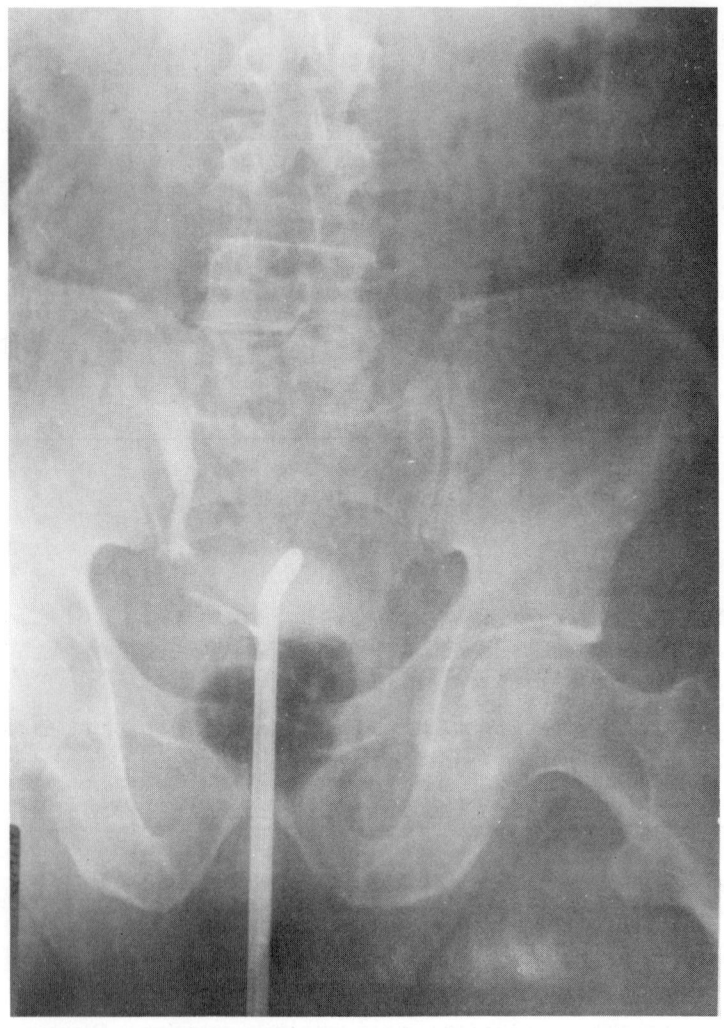

FIG. 32.2: Retrograde ureteropyelogram confirming filling defect, right lower ureter.

desquamated cells from the tumor may even resemble normal cells. In this situation, only a positive finding would be helpful in the differential diagnosis.

4. (D) The treatment for tumors of the ureter or pelvis is nephroureterectomy, including a cuff of bladder. There is a high degree of recurrence in the distal ureter, if total ureterectomy is not performed for these neoplasms.

5. (D) Riches has reported a 41% 5-year survival rate in patients with primary ureteral tumors. Bloom, et al., reported a 43% overall 5-year survival rate.

REFERENCES

1. Riches EW, Griffith IH, and Thackeray AC: New growth of the kidney and ureter. Brit J Urol 23:297, 1951.

2. Bloom NA, Vidone RA, and Litton B: Primary carcinoma of the ureter: A report of 102 cases. J Urol 103:590, 1970.

CASE 33: 53-YEAR-OLD FEMALE WITH ABDOMINAL PAIN

HISTORY

A 53-year-old white female was admitted with a chief complaint of midabdominal and right lower back pain. She was well until the day prior to admission, when she developed these symptoms. On the day of admission, she vomited once, and had several syncopal episodes. She was seen in the emergency room, and admitted immediately.

PHYSICAL EXAMINATION

BP 130/80. Pulse 110 regular. There was a large, tender mass in the right upper quadrant. Remainder of the physical examination was within normal limits.

LABORATORY DATA

Hemoglobin 8gm%. Hematocrit 25%. WBC 12,700 with 80 segs. Chemical profile was entirely within normal limits. Urinalysis revealed 8-12 WBCs per high power field. No RBCs were seen. Urine culture showed no growth.

CLINICAL COURSE

The patient was admitted to the medical service with a tentative diagnosis of a bleeding aneurysm. An aortogram was performed immediately. On this examination, it was noted that there was a tumor in the lower pole of the right kidney, with abnormal vasculature and aneurysm formation outside the renal capsule (Fig. 33.1). A preoperative diagnosis of angiomyolipoma of the kidney was made, and she was immediately taken to the OR. The abdomen was explored, and a large hematoma of the right flank was found secondary to a tumor at the lower pole of the kidney. A radical nephrectomy was performed. Postoperative course was uneventful, and she was discharged on the 10th postoperative day. After several transfusions, her hemoglobin was 10.3 gm% and Hct. 32%.

QUESTIONS

1. Angiomyolipoma may be associated with:
    A. Tuberculosis
    B. Multiple endocrine tumors
    C. Tuberous sclerosis
    D. Myelofibrosis

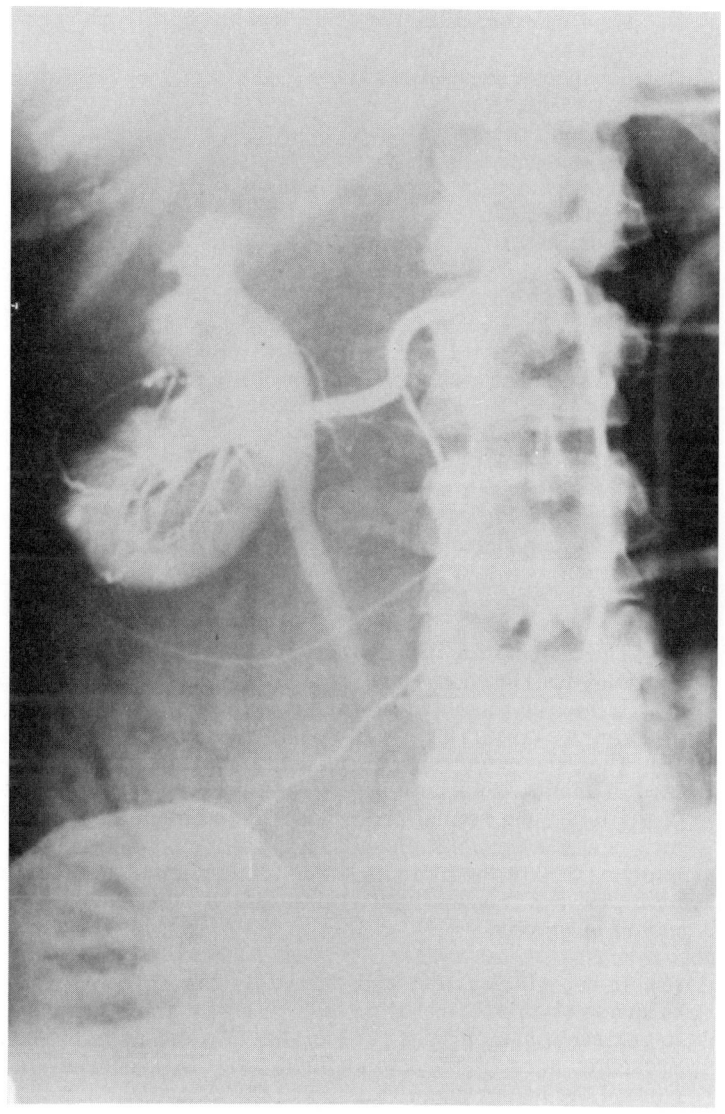

FIG. 33.1: Right renal angiogram showing mass in right kidney with small aneurysm formation indicative of angiomyolipoma.

2. Which of the following are not in the symptom complex of tuberous sclerosis?
   A. Mental retardation
   B. Epilepsy
   C. Sebaceous adenomas of face
   D. Retinal phacomas
   E. Cerebellar tumors

3. What percentage of angiomyolipomas will present with hemorrhage?
   A. Less than 10%
   B. 10-20%
   C. 20-30%
   D. Over 50%

4. Regarding angiomyolipoma, which of the following findings apply?
   A. Middle-aged female
   B. Sudden flank or abdominal pain
   C. Palpable mass which is tender
   D. Angiographic evidence of a vascular renal tumor
   E. All of the above

ANSWERS AND DISCUSSION

1. (C) The association of renal tumors with tuberous sclerosis has been known for many years, and has made this lesion clinically important to the urologist.

2. (E) Tuberous sclerosis is a hereditary disease characterized by mental retardation, epilepsy, sebaceous adenomas of the face, and retinal phacomas. Renal angiolipomatosis may occur in association with this disease complex in as many as 80% of the patients. The tumors may be single or multiple, and frequently are bilateral. It occurs more commonly in women.

3. (C) In reported series, approximately 25% of patients show evidence of an extrarenal pattern with symptoms referable to perirenal hemorrhage. When this occurs, as in the case presented here, nephrectomy invariably is necessary to control the hemorrhage.

4. (E) Renal angiomyolipoma always should be considered when a middle-aged woman complains of fairly sudden flank or abdominal pains, with a tender, palpable mass in the kidney, and a vascular renal tumor on angiography.

REFERENCES

1. Price EB and Mostofi FK: Symptomatic angiomyolipoma of the kidney. Cancer 18:761-774, 1965.

2. Seshanarayana K and Keats TE: Angiomyolipoma of the kidney: Diagnostic roentgenographic findings. Am J Roentgen 104:332-334, 1968.

3. Moudad IM, et al.: Symptomatic renal angiomyolipoma: Report of 8 cases, 2 with spontaneous rupture. J Urol 119: 684, 1978.

CASE 34: 65-YEAR-OLD MALE WITH CHEST MASS

HISTORY

A 65-year-old male was admitted to the hospital because a "coin lesion" was found in the left upper lobe of his lung on a routine chest x-ray. He denied cough or pain. There were no respiratory symptoms, and, in fact, he stated he never felt better in his life. He had nocturia once nightly, but denied any other urinary symptoms. There was no history of smoking, exposure to tuberculosis, pneumonia, or pleurisy. He had diabetes mellitus for the past 3 years, and was on Tolinase 250/mg b.i.d. with good control.

PHYSICAL EXAMINATION

Blood pressure 170/90. Heart and chest normal. The abdomen was quite obese, but there were no masses palpable. The remainder of the physical examination was unremarkable.

LABORATORY DATA

Urine analysis 4-8 WBC per high power field. No RBCs seen. Hemoglobin 13 gm%. Hematocrit 38%. Blood urea nitrogen 16 mg%. Creatinine 0.7mg%. Chemical profile on several occasions normal. Urine cytology was negative for malignant cells. Pulmonary function studies revealed a mild obstructive airway disease. EKG within normal limits. Chest x-ray showed a left upper lobe mass that was sharply marginated (Fig. 34.1).

An intravenous urogram revealed a mass in the upper lobe of the left kidney, and infusion nephrotomography confirmed the presence of the mass (Fig. 34.2). Barium enema and GI series were normal.

QUESTIONS

1. The next investigative procedure for the patient should be:
   A. Left retrograde
   B. Left thoractomy
   C. Left nephrectomy
   D. Renal angiography
   E. Sonography

2. The most common site of metastases for renal cell tumor is:
   A. Liver
   B. Regional lymph nodes

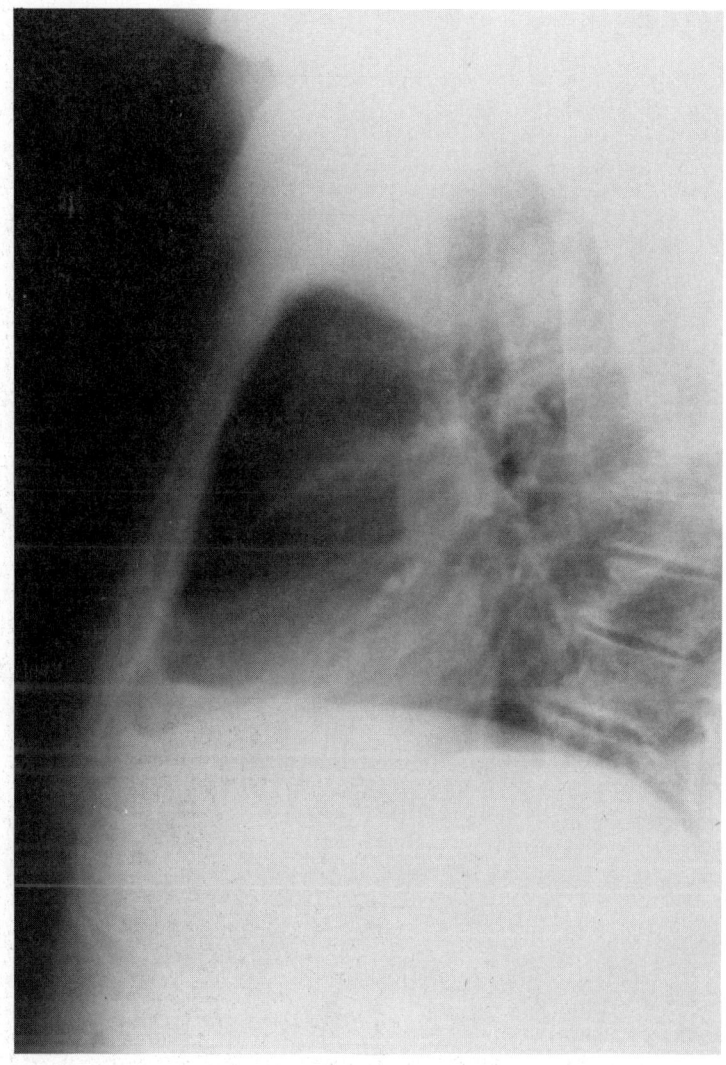

FIG. 34.1: Chest x-ray showing silver dollar-sized coin lesion in upper lobe on left.

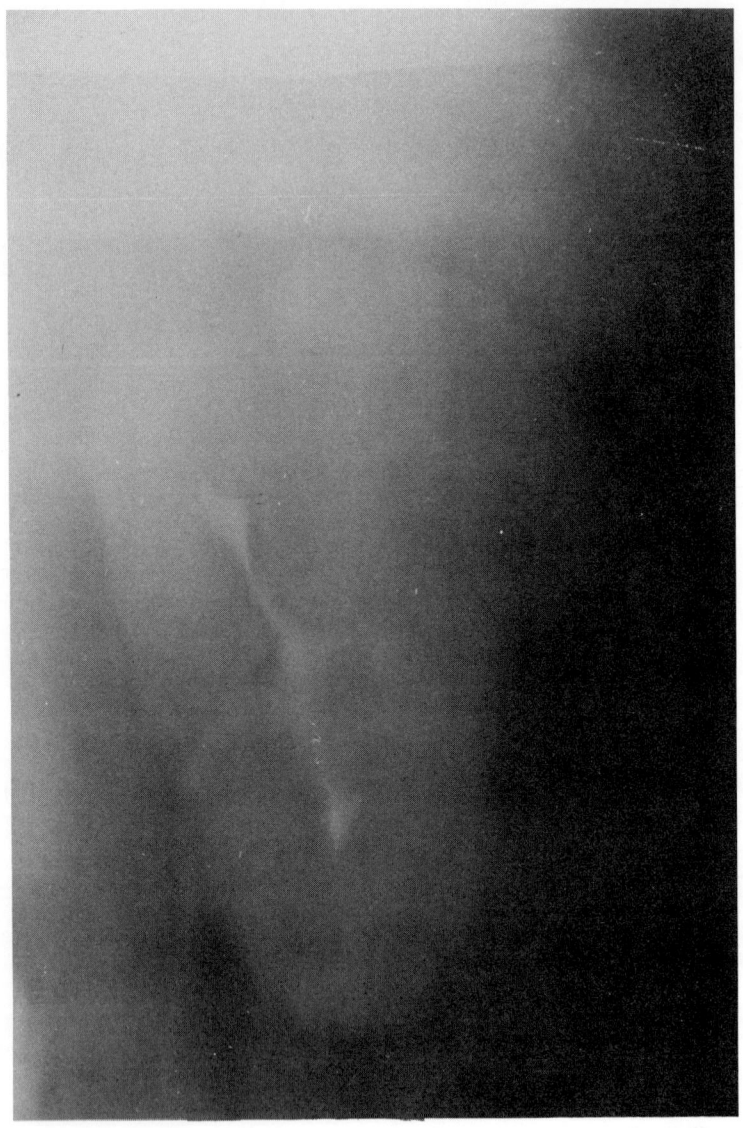

FIG. 34.2: Intravenous urogram showing large mass in upper pole of left kidney.

Renal Tumors

    C. Lung
    D. Renal vein
    E. Brain

3. The most common tumor metastatic to the kidney is:
    A. Stomach
    B. Colon
    C. Lung
    D. Prostate
    E. Bladder

4. What percentage of renal adenocarcinoma will show evidence of metastases when first seen?
    A. 10%
    B. 20%
    C. 30%
    D. 40%
    E. 50%

CLINICAL COURSE

Sonography showed a solid mass. Renal arteriography was carried out, which revealed a typical renal carcinoma in the upper pole of the left kidney (Fig. 34.3). He also underwent bronchoscopy with bronchial washings and, although these were histologically inconclusive, it was felt that he probably had a clear cell carcinoma with metastases to the lung.

5. Proper therapy for the above would be:
    A. Chemotherapy only
    B. Radical nephrectomy followed by observation for possible disappearance of metastases
    C. Radical nephrectomy and upper lobe lobectomy
    D. Nothing, since all is hopeless

6. The expected 5-year survival rate for patient with clear cell carcinoma with a solitary metastatic nodule is:
    A. Less than 10%
    B. 20%
    C. 34%
    D. 44%
    E. 50%

The patient underwent a left radical nephrectomy, and had a totally uneventful postoperative course. Pathology report was clear cell carcinoma of the kidney. There was no evidence of renal vein involvement; 21 nodes were examined for tumor, and were found to be negative.

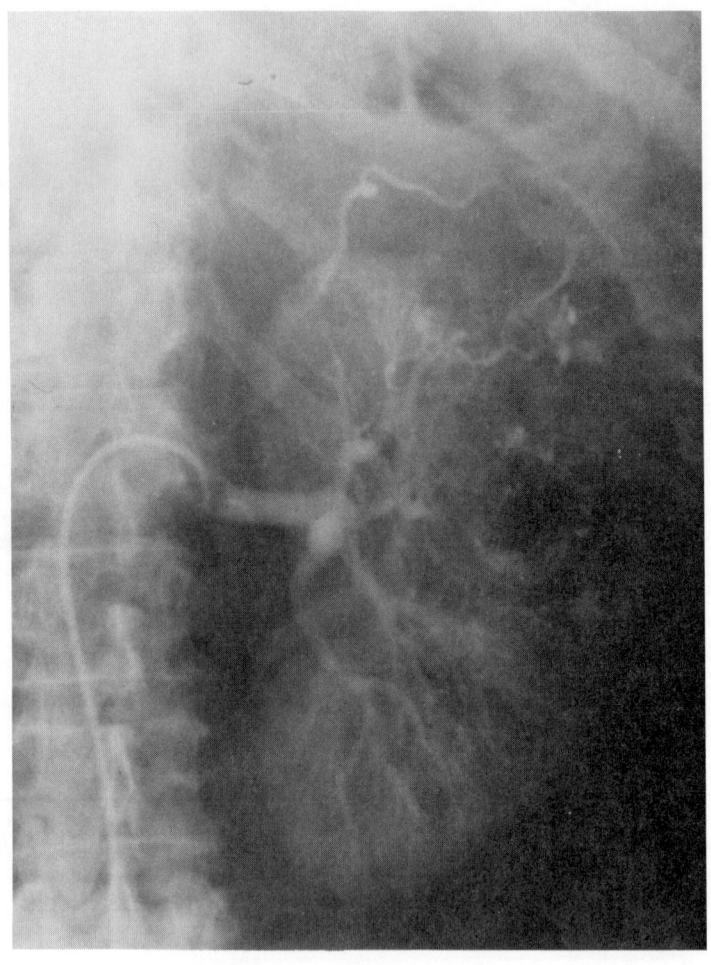

FIG. 34.3A: Left renal angiogram showing typical angiographic pattern of renal cell carcinoma (see Fig. 34.3B).

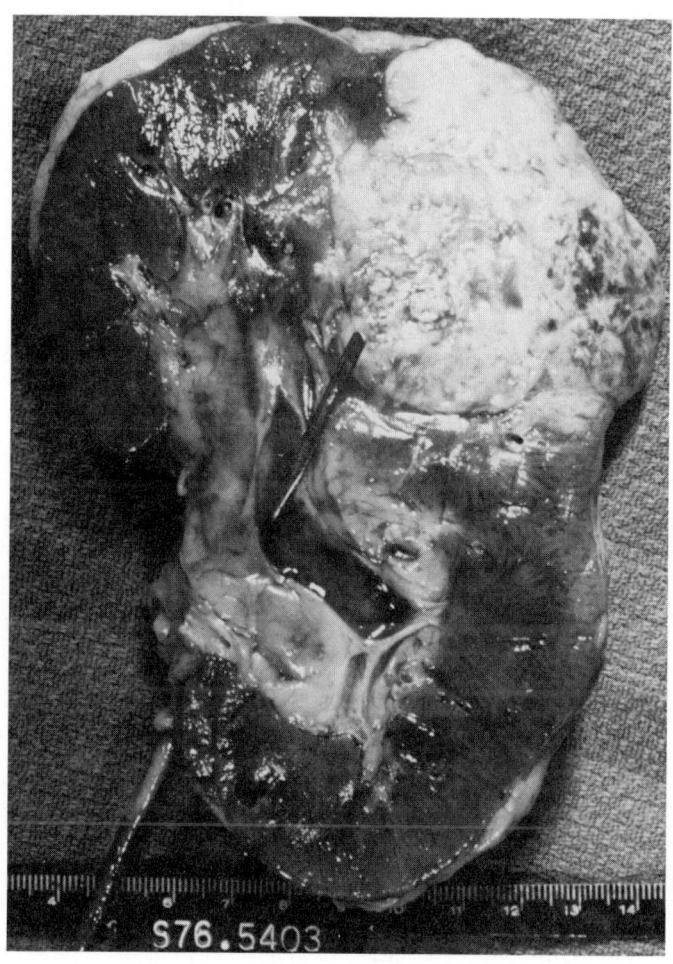

FIG. 34.3B: Gross pathology of the same specimen.

He was readmitted to the hospital 6 weeks later. The chest x-ray had not changed appreciably. He underwent left thoracotomy at that time. There was no evidence of metastatic disease in the mediastinum, and a left lobe lobectomy was performed. He made an uneventful recovery. Pathology report of the lung lesion was bronchial adenoma carcinoid type.

The patient has been followed for 18 months since that time, and is apparently free of metastases.

ANSWERS AND DISCUSSION

1. (E) After a mass is located on intravenous urography, the next step in diagnosis should be sonography. If this shows a solid mass, as occurred in this case, then one should proceed directly to renal angiography. If this proves to be a tumor, then surgery would be indicated. If there is no evidence of metastatic disease, in the presence of a solitary metastatic lesion, one would generally excise both lesions in the hope of a cure.

2. (C) In the series of the Armed Forces Institute of Pathology, pulmonary metastases comprised 55.9% of all metastatic lesions. This was followed by lymph nodes (38.1%), liver (35.0%), bones (33.1%), adrenal (18.8%).

3. (C) Pulmonary carcinoma has been found to be the most common tumor metastatic to the kidney in the British Tumor Registry. This diagnosis is generally made at postmortem examination, however.

4. (C) In the New York Hospital series reported by Middleton, 141 of 503 cases (28.0%) had multiple metastatic lesions when first seen, and 8 cases (1.6%) had only solitary metastases. Other series also report an incidence in the range of 30%.

5. (C) Barney and Churchill reported the first case in which a patient underwent both nephrectomy and excision of a solitary pulmonary metastasis. Their patient lived 23 years and died of other causes. This case has prompted other surgeons to treat cases of solitary metastasis in a similar manner as well. Sometimes nephrectomy is done, with the hope of regression of multiple metastases. In Middleton's series, 33 of 141 patients had nephrectomy for multiple metastases. There was no significant increase in survival in these patients, however.

6. (C) In Middleton's review of the literature, 59 patients had been reported who underwent nephrectomy and removal of a solitary metastatic lesion. Of these, 45% survived 3 years, and 34% survived 5 years. These survival rates are close to those following nephrectomy in the absence of apparent metastatic disease.

REFERENCES

1. Barney JD and Churchill EJ: Adenocarcinoma of the kidney with metastasis to the lung; cured by nephrectomy and lobectomy. J Urol 42:269, 1939.

2. Middleton RG: Surgery for metastatic renal cell carcinoma. J Urol 97:973, 1967.

3. Johnson DE, Kaesler KE, and Samuels ML: Is nephrectomy justified in patient with metastatic renal carcinoma? J Urol 114:27-29, 1975.

CASE 35: 8-YEAR-OLD BOY WITH AN ABDOMINAL MASS

HISTORY

This 8-year-old child was admitted when his pediatrician found a large abdominal mass on a routine physical examination. He had weighed 8 pounds at birth and had a normal growth and development. His only significant history was enuresis. There was no gross hematuria or flank pain.

PHYSICAL EXAMINATION

Blood pressure 130/90. Pulse 90. Temp 37.1C°. The abdomen was distended, and veins were prominent. There was a mass in the right upper quadrant. It was approximately 15 x 10cm in size, and extended across the midline. It was very hard and irregular, but movable. The remainder of the examination was normal.

LABORATORY DATA

Hematocrit on admission, 31%. CPK, 588 units. LDH, 428 units. Urinalysis, electrolytes, glucose, and entire chemical profile, other than the above, were all within normal limits.

CLINICAL COURSE

An intravenous urogram revealed a large mass in the lower pole of the right kidney with a hydronephrotic upper pole segment (Fig. 35.1).

Ultrasonography showed this mass to be solid, but areas of hemorrhage and necrosis were apparent within it. Renal angiography and inferior vena cavagraphy also were performed, and revealed marked neovascularity of the tumor, with arteriovenous shunting, as well as external compression of the vena cava by the mass (Fig. 35.2 and 35.3). Liver and spleen scans were normal. Lung tomograms showed no evidence of pulmonary metastasis. Metastatic survey showed no evidence of metastasis. The patient was treated with vincristine for one week preoperatively, but showed little response. A right radical nephrectomy was performed, along with resection of a portion of the vena cava. The child made an uneventful recovery.

Pathology revealed a Wilms' tumor, which was of the "blastoma type," occupying most of the kidney. The renal capsule, Gerota's fascia, lymph nodes, renal vein, and all lines of resection were

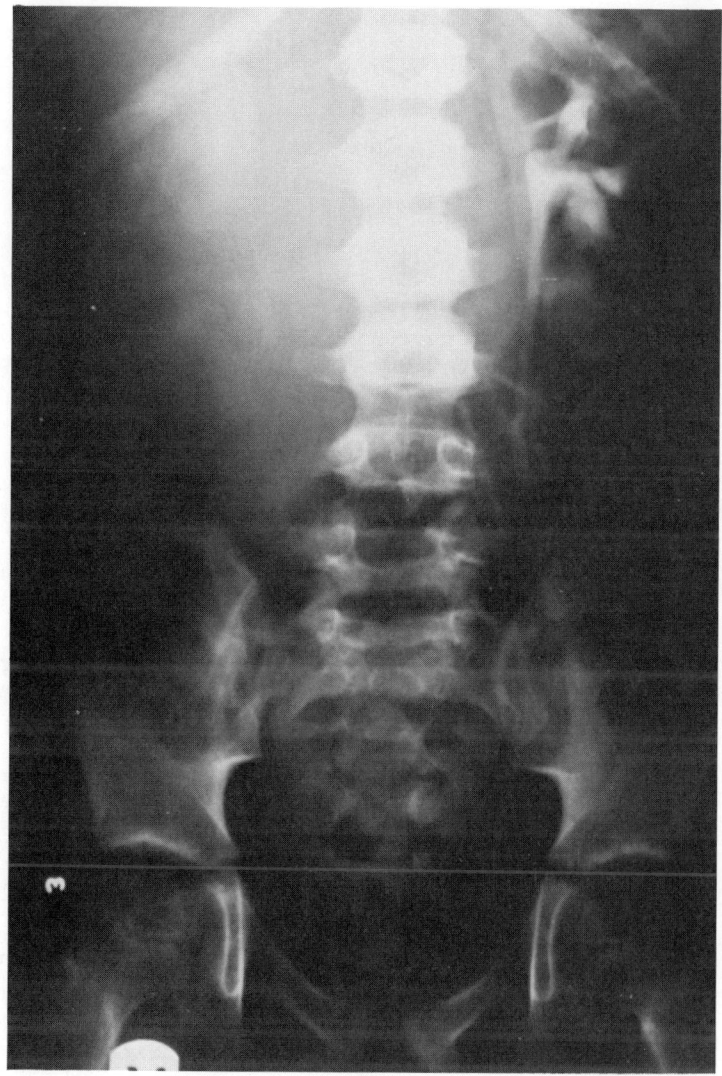

FIG. 35.1: Intravenous urogram showing Wilms' tumor of lower pole of kidney with hydronephrotic upper pole segment.

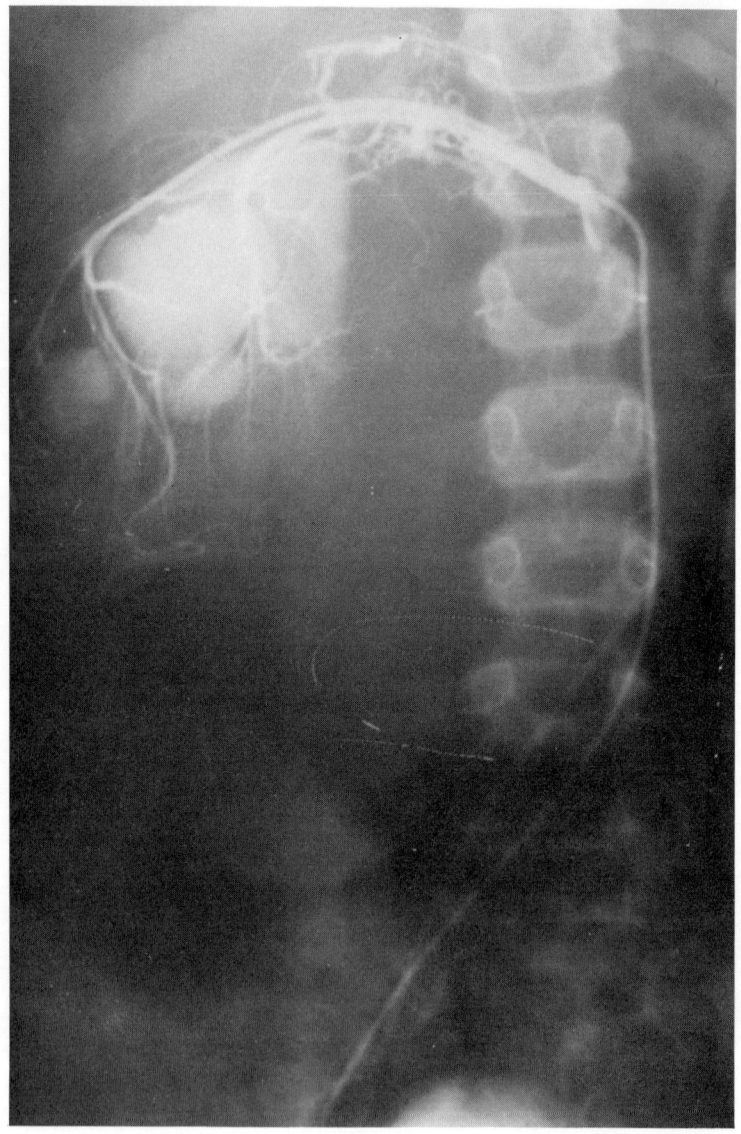

FIG. 35.2: Renal angiogram showing neovascularity of large lower pole tumor.

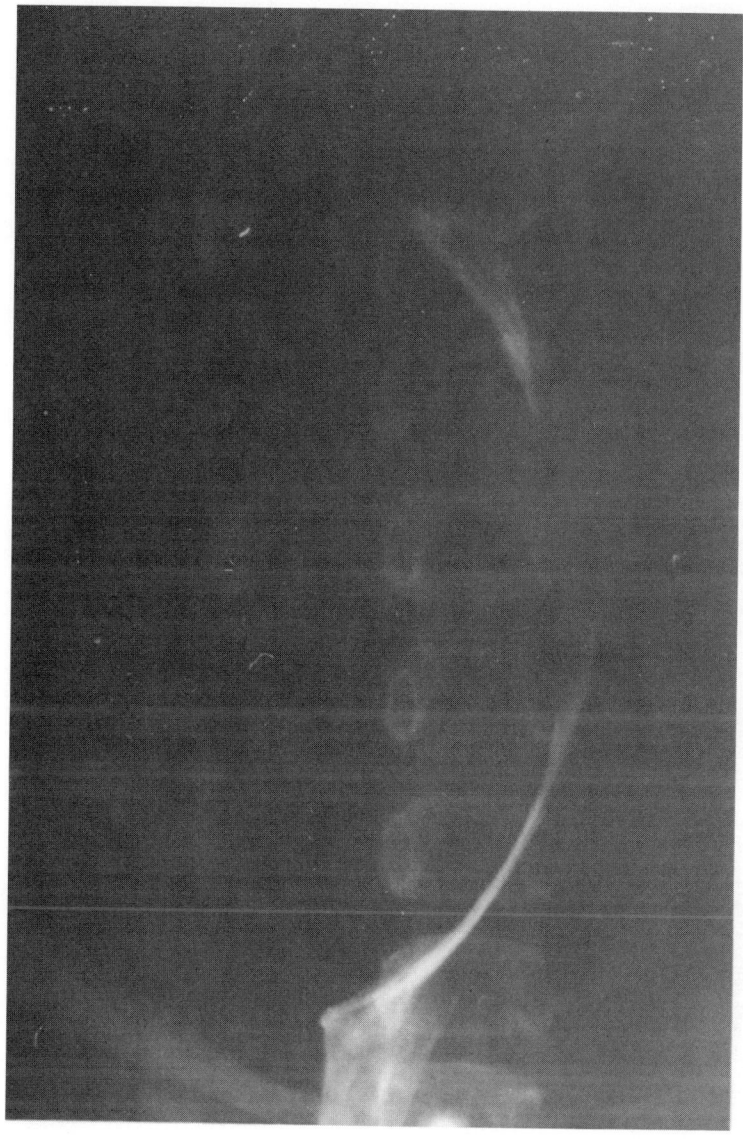

FIG. 35.3: Inferior vena cavagram. The vena cava is shifted markedly by external compression.

free of tumor. The vena cava, which was resected, was free of tumor. The child has been followed for 8 months, and apparently is free of disease.

QUESTIONS

1. Nonvisualization of the kidney on excretory urography in a child is indicative of:
   A. Hydronephrotic kidney
   B. Wilms' tumor
   C. Agenesis of the kidney
   D. All of the above
   E. A & C

2. The chemotherapeutic drug of choice in Wilms' tumor is:
   A. Vincristine
   B. 5-Fluorouracil
   C. Actinomycin D
   D. Bleomycin
   E. A & C

3. Fetal renal hamartoma, which is benign, closely resembles:
   A. Neuroblastoma
   B. Orchioblastoma
   C. Wilms' tumor
   D. Renal cell carcinoma
   E. Liposarcoma

4. A small but significant association has been found between Wilms' tumor and:
   A. Aniridia
   B. Anosmia
   C. Alexia
   D. Ataxia

5. The treatment of choice for Stage I Wilms' tumor (confined to the kidney) is:
   A. Nephrectomy
   B. Nephrectomy and radiation
   C. Nephrectomy and actinomycin D
   D. Nephrectomy, actinomycin D and vincristine
   E. Nephrectomy, radiotherapy and actinomycin

ANSWERS AND DISCUSSION

1. (D) A renal mass, present on physical examination and with no visualization on excretory urography, in general, will indicate a hydronephrotic kidney. However 10-20% of Wilms'

Renal Tumors   Case 35/ 183

tumors will show nonvisualization on intravenous urography. An extensive tumor may invade the pelvis and ureter, and cause complete obstruction, resulting in nonvisualization. It also may invade the renal vein, producing nonfunction in the kidney. With large dose urography, there generally will be some evidence of excretion in the obstructed kidney, making the differential diagnosis easier. Of course, agenesis of the kidney also will show nonvisualization.

2. (E) Both vincristine and actinomycin D have been shown to be effective in Wilms' tumor, and are used extensively for treatment in all stages.

3. (C) Fetal renal hamartoma or congenital mesoblastic nephroma are the most common renal tumors seen in the first few weeks of life. The most common presenting symptom is an abdominal mass. At times, it is confused with Wilms' tumor, but is distinguishable easily from both by its gross and histologic appearance. The only treatment is nephrectomy.

4. (A) Aniridia is only one of the congenital anomalies sometimes associated with Wilms' tumor. Others are hemihypertrophy, visceral cytomegaly, hamartomas, and genitourinary tract anomalies. The great majority of patients with Wilms' tumor do not have these anomalies.

5. (D) The National Wilms' Tumor Study recommends nephrectomy, plus actinomycin D and vincristine. The role of radiotherapy, at the time of this writing, has not been advocated for Stage I disease.

REFERENCE

1. Gilchrist GS and Kelalis PP: Chapter 24A. In: Clinical Pediatric Urology, Kelalis PP and King LR (eds.), W.B. Saunders Company, Philadelphia, 1976, p. 896.

CASE 36: 40-YEAR-OLD MALE WITH RIGHT RENAL COLIC

HISTORY

A 40-year-old male was seen because of right renal colic of several hours duration, which subsided spontaneously. There was no past history of calculus disease, nor was there a family history of calculus disease. He denied gross hematuria, chills, or fever. He was seen several days after the episode of hematuria and was asymptomatic. He had not passed a stone in the interim.

PHYSICAL EXAMINATION

Blood pressure, pulse, and respiration were normal. There were no palpable abdominal masses. There was no CVA tenderness.

LABORATORY DATA

Urine analysis was normal; there were no RBCs present. CBC and blood urea nitrogen were normal. Intravenous urogram showed no evidence of calculi, and the right collecting system and ureter were normal. On the lateral border of the left kidney, there was a radiolucent mass measuring approximately 5 cm in diameter (Fig. 36.1).

QUESTIONS

1. The next step in the evaluation of this patient should be:
   A. Infusion nephrotomography
   B. Renal sonography
   C. Renal angiography
   D. Exploration of the kidney

2. Radiolucent renal masses may be indicative of:
   A. Solitary renal cyst
   B. Clear cell carcinoma
   C. Renal carbuncle
   D. Hamartoma of kidney
   E. All of the above

3. The differentiation of simple renal cyst vs. pyelogenic cyst can be made on:
   A. Intravenous urography
   B. Retrograde pyelogram
   C. Nephrotomogram
   D. Sonography

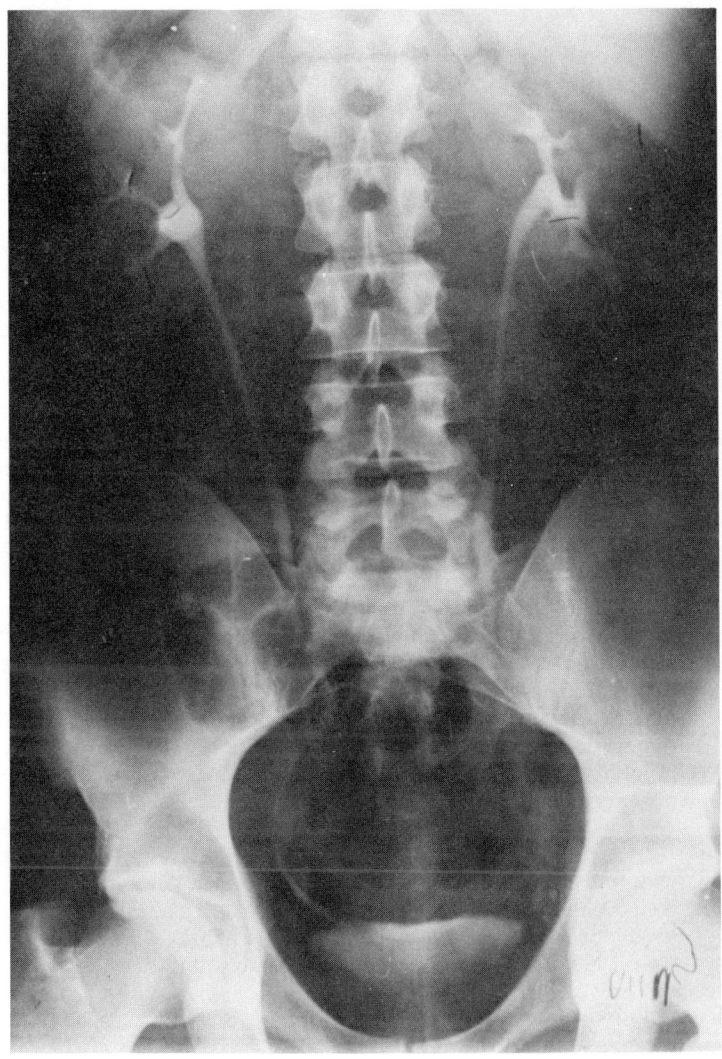

FIG. 36.1: Intravenous urogram showing radiolucent mass on lateral border of left kidney.

Renal sonography was performed next, and this revealed a cystic mass in the lateral border of the left kidney measuring 5.5cm (Fig. 36.2).

4. Following this procedure, one would perform:
    A. Renal exploration
    B. Left renal angiography
    C. Infusion nephrotomography
    D. Renal cyst puncture
    E. Observation only

5. What percentage of apparently benign renal cysts will show neoplasm in the cyst wall?
    A. 10-20%
    B. 20-30%
    C. 30-40%
    D. Less than 5%

A renal cyst puncture was performed, and 20cc of clear, straw-colored fluid was aspirated. Cytology of the fluid failed to show any evidence of abnormal cells.

ANSWERS AND DISCUSSION

1. (B) At our Institution, in this situation, the next step is that sonography is performed. Next, if the mass is definitely solid, then angiography is done. If it appears to be definitely cystic, as in this case, needle aspiration is performed with sonographic control. If there is any question, then we would proceed to angiography. In the presence of a clear fluid with no abnormal cells and normal chemistry, we feel there is no necessity to evaluate further.

2. (E) All of the foregoing possibilities should be considered in the differential diagnosis of radiolucent masses. Most of those mentioned would show a solid mass, or at least some evidence of echoes on sonography. Further differentiation would have to be carried out by angiography and surgery.

3. (B) Pyelogenic cyst would be shown to be contiguous with the collecting system on retrograde pyelography, and the cyst cavity would fill with contrast material. A simple renal cyst would show only as a mass and pressure defect on retrograde pyelogram.

4. (D) As previously stated, if sonography shows a cystic mass, with no evidence of echoes, then renal cyst puncture can be

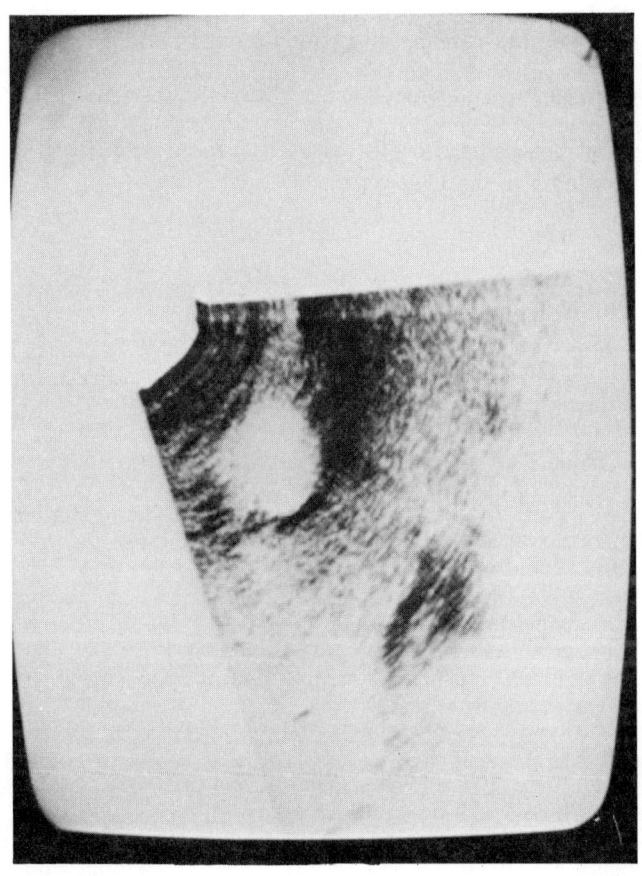

FIG. 36.2: Nephrosonography. There is a large cystic mass present.

performed. We have had minimal complications following this course of investigation of the patient.

5. (D) Tumor in the wall of what appears to be a benign cyst occurs in less than 5% of cases, probably less than 1% or 2%. One would expect at least some evidence of blood to be present within the cyst fluid, as well as to have some evidence of malignancy on cytologic examination.

See Case 39 for references and additional questions.

CASE 37: 8-MONTH-OLD CHILD WITH FEVER, WEIGHT LOSS AND SEPSIS

HISTORY

An 8-month-old child was admitted to the hospital with fever, weight loss, and sepsis. Urine smear in the emergency room revealed gram negative rods. The child appeared very acutely ill, and was given 15mg of gentamycin.

PHYSICAL EXAMINATION

An acutely ill child who appeared quite dehydrated; heart and chest were normal; there were no abdominal masses; genitals were normal.

LABORATORY DATA

Urinalysis revealed many WBCs, and smear showed many gram negative rods. Sodium 127mEq/l. Potassium 6.9mEq/l. Chloride 89mEq/l CO_2 2mEq/l.   Blood urea nitrogen 90mg on admission. Urine culture later grew out E. coli.

CLINICAL COURSE

The child was treated with intravenous fluids, and no further antibiotics were given. Over the next 12 hours, there was no urinary output.

The child was taken to the cystoscopy room, a catheter passed to the left renal pelvis, and a hydronephrotic drip obtained. A catheter could be passed only 7cm up the right ureter, and retrograde injection failed to fill the renal pelvis. There was a question of extravasation. A percutaneous right nephrostogram was performed. This catheter never drained urine; so two days later, the right kidney was explored with the intent of performing a nephrostomy. A multicystic kidney was found, and a nephrectomy performed (Fig. 37.1).

The left ureteral catheter continued to drain urine, and the blood urea nitrogen fell to 25mg%, and creatinine to 1.7mg%. Ureteropelvic junction obstruction on the right was present, and one week later this kidney was explored. A very small pelvis was found, and a ureterocalycostomy was performed, and a nephrostomy left in place.

Ten days later, nephrostogram showed no evidence of obstruction, and the tube was removed. The child made an uneventful recovery.

See Case 39 for references and questions.

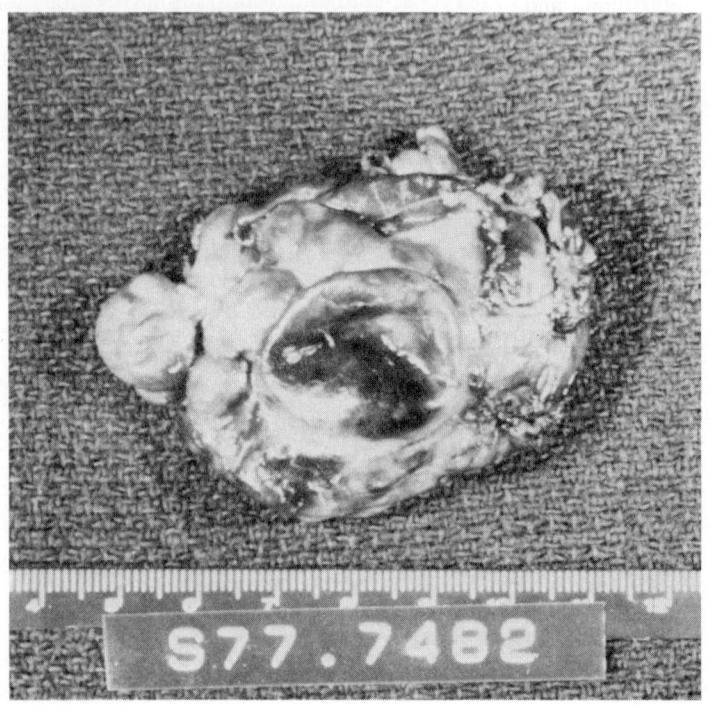

FIG. 37.1: Multicystic kidney.

CASE 38: 42-YEAR-OLD MALE WITH GROSS HEMATURIA

HISTORY

A 42-year-old male was seen in the emergency room because of gross total painless hematuria and left flank pain, which had been present for the past several hours. There was no previous history of urinary tract disease. He denied fever or chills, frequency, urgency, or dysuria. There was no family history of renal disease.

PHYSICAL EXAMINATION

Blood pressure 130/80. Heart and lungs were normal. There were no masses palpable abdominally. There was moderate right CVA tenderness. Genitalia and rectal examination were normal.

LABORATORY DATA

Urinalysis revealed many RBCs per high power field, no WBCs. Urine culture showed no growth. Blood urea nitrogen 18mg%, creatinine 1.0mg%, CBC normal. Plain film of the abdomen revealed a tiny calculus in the distal ureter, and intravenous urogram revealed delayed excretion on the left with hydroureteronephrosis down to the area of the aforementioned calcification. There was evidence of bilateral renal masses.

CLINICAL COURSE

The patient was treated with analgesics, and passed a small calculus within 24 hours. Infusion tomography was performed, and showed typical signs of polycystic renal disease (Fig. 38.1). The patient again stated there was no family history of renal disease. He was apprised of the situation and diagnosis, and advised to have semiannual urologic checkups, as well as to have his entire immediate family investigated urologically.

See Case 39 for questions and references.

192/ Case 38 Renal Tumors

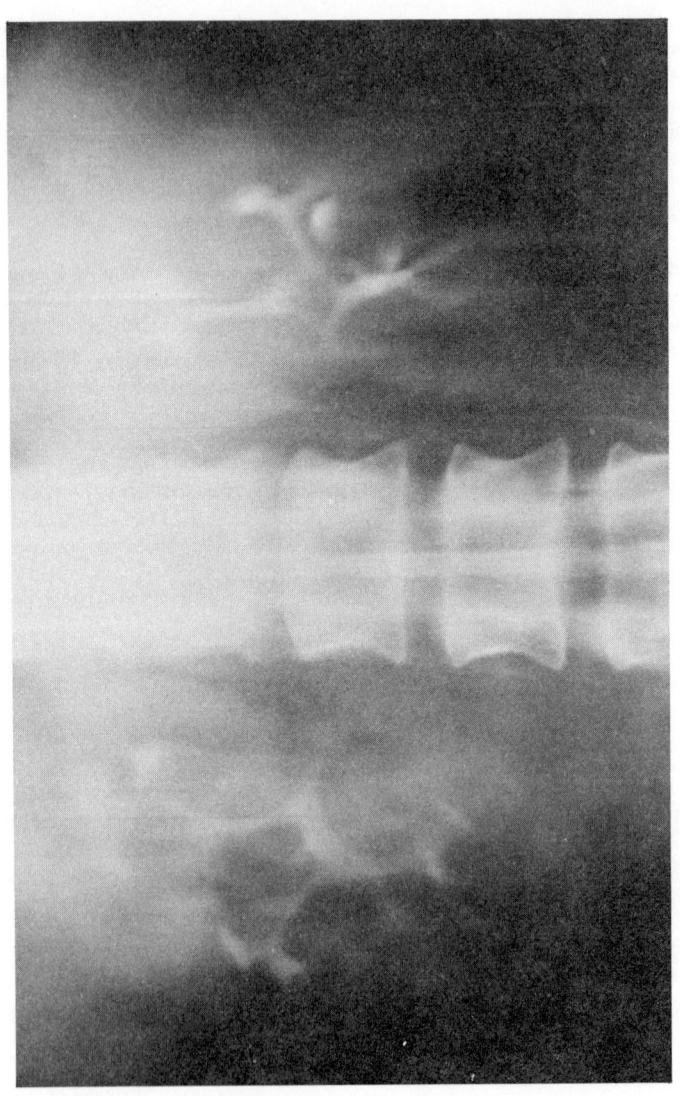

FIG. 38.1: Infusion tomography showing typical polycystic renal disease.

CASE 39: 68-YEAR-OLD MALE WITH DIFFICULTY VOIDING

HISTORY

A 68-year-old male was seen because of difficulty voiding. He complained of having to strain to urinate, as well as nocturia 3 to 4 times, and a slow urinary stream. Two months prior, he had had an anterior resection for adenocarcinoma of the rectosigmoid. He denied urinary symptoms prior to this surgery. Past medical history was unremarkable.

PHYSICAL EXAMINATION

Blood pressure, 150/90. Heart and chest within normal limits. There was a left paramedian, well-healed scar. No masses were palpable abdominally. External genitalia were normal. Rectal examination revealed only a slightly enlarged, benign prostate. The bulbocavernosus reflex showed a poor response.

LABORATORY DATA

Urinalysis normal. Urine culture showed no growth. CBC normal. Blood urea nitrogen 15mg%, creatinine 0.8mg%. An intravenous urogram and tomography revealed a left peripelvic cyst (Fig. 39.1), but was otherwise normal.

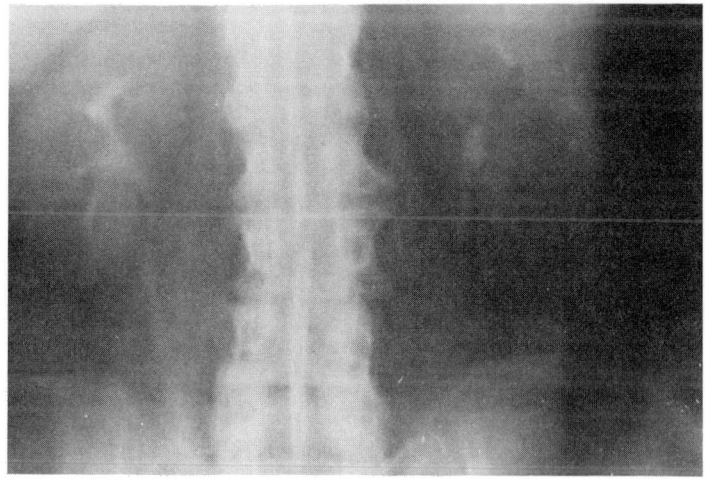

FIG. 39.1: Intravenous urogram with tomography showing a left parapelvic cyst.

There was a large postvoid residual urine. Catheterized residual was 200cc and a cystometrogram revealed a flat curve with no proprioception, with 700cc in the bladder (Fig. 39.2A). Sonography confirmed the presence of a left peripelvic cyst (Fig. 39.3).

CLINICAL COURSE

Cystoscopy was performed, and revealed only a mildly trabeculated bladder. The prostate was not obstructed completely.

The patient was placed on bethanechol 25mg q.i.d., which subsequently was increased to 50mg q.i.d. His symptoms improved dramatically. A repeat cystometrogram showed a normal curve. He continued on this medication, and a repeat postvoid residual several months later was only 30cc (see Fig. 39.2B).

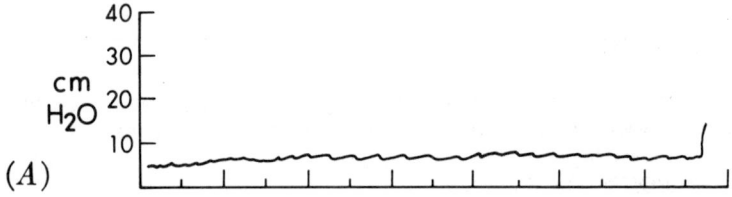

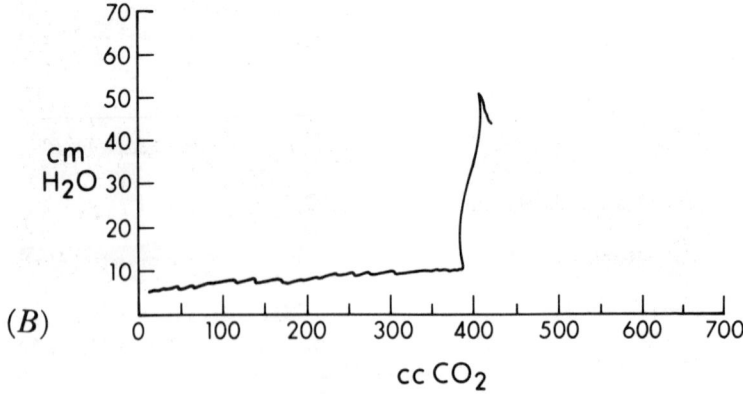

FIG. 39.2: (A) Cystometrogram prior to initiation of treatment
(B) Cystometrogram 6 weeks after bethanechol 50 mg q.i.d.

Renal Tumors

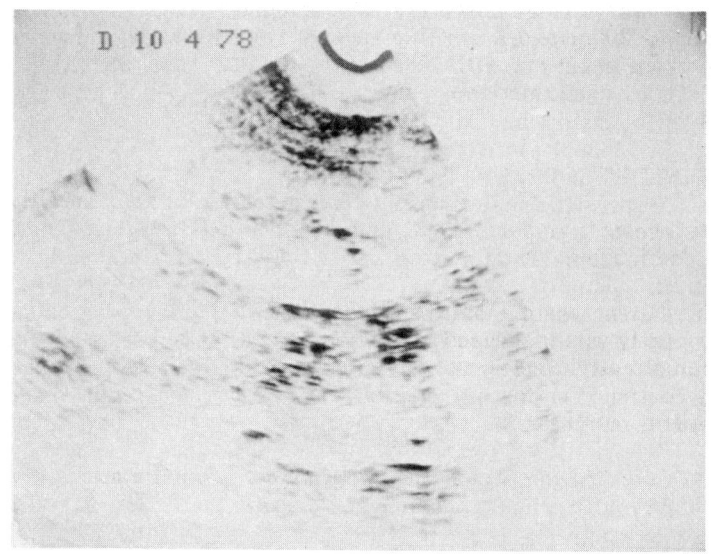

FIG. 39.3: Sonography of left parapelvic cyst.

QUESTIONS: CASES 36-39

1. All of the following are true in relation to multicystic kidney, except:
   A. It is almost always unilateral
   B. It is inherited by an autosomal recessive trait
   C. It is characterized by an irregular lobulated mass of cysts
   D. The ureter is usually atretic or absent

2. The best method of diagnosis of a multicystic kidney is:
   A. Intravenous urogram
   B. Renal angiography
   C. Retrograde ureteropyelogram
   D. Renal sonography
   E. Surgical exploration

3. Renal dysplasia can be found in which of the following?
   A. Ureterocele with duplication
   B. Ureteropelvic junction obstruction
   C. Multicystic kidney
   D. Congenital reflux
   E. All of the above

4. Multiple renal cysts are characterized by:
   A. Microhematuria
   B. Renal failure
   C. Abdominal pain
   D. Asymptomatic
   E. Inherited disorder

5. Polycystic renal disease is characterized by all of the above, except:
   A. Microhematuria
   B. Renal failure
   C. Autosomal dominant inheritance
   D. Autosomal recessive inheritance
   E. Adult onset

(T)RUE OR (F)ALSE:

6. Calcification around the periphery of a renal mass is indicative of renal cyst in 95% of cases.

7. Central, stippled calcification within a renal mass indicates neoplasm.

8. Parapelvic cysts are thought to be lymphatic in origin.

9. Arteriography often is necessary in the diagnosis of polycystic renal disease.

ANSWERS AND DISCUSSION: CASES 36-39

1. (B) Multicystic kidney is not an inherited disease. Almost always, it is unilateral and, when bilateral, it is fatal, since there is no functioning tissue present. It is a mass of cysts with little or no recognizable renal parenchyma present. The prevailing theory for its development is faulty union of the nephron and collecting system. It usually is discovered as an irregular mass in the newborn or infant.

2. (D) Intravenous urogram will show only nonvisualization of the affected area and can be due to hydronephrosis, tumor, or agenesis. Renal angiography may make the diagnosis, but is not the best method, since this can be dangerous in a newborn or infant. Retrograde studies would be impossible because of the absent or atretic ureter, and would not differentiate this lesion from agenesis. Renal sonography is almost pathognomonic. The decision for surgery would depend on the size of the cystic changes, as well as symptoms.

Renal Tumors

3. (E) In renal dysplasia, the renal parenchyma is totally disorganized. There is fetal type of renal parenchyma present with tubular and glomerular cysts seen. Metaplastic areas of cartilage may be seen as well. These changes are seen in conditions where obstruction or reflux begin in early fetal life. It also may be seen in multicystic kidney.

4. (D) Multiple renal cysts are just an extension of solitary renal cystic disease and, generally, are asymptomatic, and found inadvertently when intravenous urography is performed for other genitourinary problems. They rarely cause hematuria, and almost never give rise to renal failure. They are differentiated from polycystic renal disease by the latter two symptoms; there is also no family history of the disorder.

5. (D) Adult type of polycystic renal disease is an autosomal, dominantly inherited disorder. Almost invariably, there is a family history present. Microhematuria, as well as gross hematuria, is a common presenting symptom. Renal failure occurs frequently, and dialysis or transplantation may become necessary.

6. (F) At one time, it was thought that peripheral calcification of a mass was pathognomonic of simple cyst. More recent studies have shown that as many as 20% of peripherally calcified lesions may be neoplastic in origin. Although most centrally, stippled-type calcifications are neoplastic in nature, a good percentage of these may be secondary to inflammatory processes.[3]

7. (F)

8. (T) One of the many theories of pathogenesis of parapelvic cysts is that they are derived from ectatic, obstructed renal lymphatics. This is substantiated by the fact that they are closely adherent to the renal pelvis, and enlarge into the renal hilum of the kidney following the course of the renal lymphatics. As the cyst grows, it compresses the renal pelvis, producing marked pelvic distortion and sometimes obstruction. This can result in difficulty in diagnosis, but when parapelvic cyst is kept in mind, the radiographic diagnosis is an easy one.

9. (T) Arteriography can be particularly helpful in the evaluation of patients with polycystic renal disease. The branches of the renal artery are stretched and elongated over the

numerous cysts present. There is renal parenchyma seen peripheral to the termination of the arteries. The absence of abnormal vessels and "tumor stain" excludes the presence of renal neoplasm. During the nephrographic phase, the typical "Swiss cheese" pattern of this disorder can be seen.

REFERENCES: CASES 36-39

1. Witten DM, Myers GH and Utz DC: Emmet's Clinical Urography, Volume 3, W.B. Saunders Company, Philadelphia, 1977, pp. 1369-1463.

2. Elkin M and Bernstein J: Cystic diseases of the kidney: Radiologic and pathologic considerations. Clin Radio 20: 65-82, Jan. 1969.

3. Daniel WW Jr, et al.: Calcified renal masses: A review of 10 years experience at the Mayo Clinic. Radiology 103:503-508, 1972.

CHAPTER VII

BLADDER TUMORS

INTRODUCTION

Bladder tumor is one of the most difficult problems confronting the urologist. Ninety-five percent of these tumors arise from transitional epithelium, the remainder from the other layers of the bladder, forming a group of rare benign and malignant tumors of smooth muscle, connective tissue, fat and neurogenic tissue.

Bladder cancer accounts for about 2% of all deaths from malignant disease. Males are afflicted about three times more frequently than females. It is generally a disease in patients beyond the age of 40, but it does occur in earlier years as well.

The etiology of bladder cancer is a fascinating area of research. It has long been known that certain work in aniline dye industries brought increased susceptibility to bladder cancer. The carcinogens found to be involved are the alpha and beta naphthylamine and benzidine. These are excreted in the urine as active carcinogens producing carcinoma only in areas with which they come into contact. Bladder cancers produced by these known carcinogens are in no way different from those seen in patients with essentially no known etiologic factor. This has been a great stimulus to research in this field. The metabolites of normal tryptophane metabolism, similar in structure to the known carcinogens, are believed to play a role in the etiology of bladder cancer. Details of this most fascinating field are beyond the scope of this discussion.

Bladder tumors generally are classified histologically as: 1) benign papilloma - a villous tumor on a narrow stalk covered with fairly normal appearing transitional epithelium, not more than about five cells thick and 2) transitional cell carcinoma which is graded 1 to 4 depending upon its differentiation or lack of it, as well as the degree of anaplasia. Metaplasia to squamous cell carcinoma generally is believed to represent the highest form of malignancy (see Case 37). Adenocarcinoma is another metaplastic variety.

Management of bladder tumors is dependent upon clinical staging of the tumor, that is, the preoperative determination of its extent. This is extremely difficult to accomplish accurately in many instances. Depth of penetration of tumors are classified according to the method of Marshall and Jewett. Techniques used to evaluate these are: cystoscopic examination; biopsy of superficial and deep portions of the tumor by transurethral resection; bimanual examination under anesthesia; and various radiographic techniques, i.e., multiple contrast cystography with and without angiography of the vesical arteries, as well as lymphangiography. The modes of therapy are surgery, radiotherapy, or chemotherapy. Surgery may include transurethral resection or simple fulguration, which can be both diagnostic as well as therapeutic, suprapubic open fulguration, segmental resection of the bladder or total cystectomy with urinary diversions. Various forms of chemotherapy are available, the most useful probably being intravesical instillation of Thio-Tepa for superficial type lesions. Bladder tumors are radiosensitive, and radiotherapy is used as both primary treatment or in conjunction with surgery and/or chemotherapy. In recent years, the use of preoperative radiotherapy has significantly increased the survival rate of bladder cancer.

Bladder Tumors   Case 40/ 201

CASE 40: 61-YEAR-OLD MALE WITH GROSS HEMATURIA

HISTORY

A 61-year-old male butcher presented with gross total painless hematuria. Past history was entirely negative.

PHYSICAL EXAMINATION: Within normal limits.

LABORATORY DATA

Urine showed gross hematuria; no WBC seen. Urine culture was negative. Intravenous urogram revealed prompt bilateral excretion with normal upper urinary tracts. The ureters were seen through their entire course and were normal. Cystoscopy revealed three small frondular tumors on narrow stalks on the dome of the bladder. These were resected transurethrally, and the pathology report was "Papilloma of urinary bladder, with no evidence of muscle invasion."

CLINICAL COURSE

Following this, the patient received a 6-week course of Thio-Tepa instillation into the bladder, 60 mgs. of Thio-Tepa in 30ccs saline being instilled once weekly. Three months later, cystoscopy again revealed a very small papillary growth on the dome of the bladder similar to those seen previously. This was fulgurated transurethrally. Four cystoscopies, over a period of 14 months, showed no evidence of recurrent tumor.

Two years after our initial visit, three papillomas were noted on the right lateral wall of the bladder. These were electrofulgurated in the office. Subsequent cystoscopies failed to reveal recurrent tumor. However, two small papillomata were fulgurated on an outpatient basis, and he has required three transurethral resections for recurrent tumors. These have never shown muscle invasion and always have been classified as bladder papillomas. There has never been evidence of metastatic disease. He has been followed for more than 20 years.

QUESTIONS

1. The most common presenting symptom of bladder tumor is:
    A. Initial hematuria
    B. Frequency of urination
    C. Gross total painless hematuria
    D. Gross total hematuria with dysuria
    E. Inadvertent finding of mirohematuria

Case 40 — Bladder Tumors

2. Which of the following are believed to be etiologic agents in bladder cancer?
   A. Cigarette smoking
   B. Schistosomiasis hematobium
   C. Tryptophan metabolites
   D. 2-naphthylamine
   E. All of the above

3. The final common pathway of the chemical carcinogen in bladder tumor is:
   A. 2-naphthylamine
   B. Tryptophan
   C. Ortho-amino-phenols
   D. Beta-glucuronidase

4. The expected 5-year survival rate for transitional cell carcinoma Grade I is:
   A. 10-20%
   B. 20-30%
   C. 30-40%
   D. 40-50%
   E. Over 75%

THE FOLLOWING STATEMENT CONSISTS OF A STATEMENT AND A REASON. ANSWER BY USING THE FOLLOWING KEY:

   A. If both statement and reason are true and related cause and effect
   B. If both statement and reason are true but not related cause and effect
   C. If the statement is true but the reason is false
   D. If the statement is false but the reason is true
   E. If both statement and reason are false

5. Cytologic examination of the urine is extremely helpful in follow-up of patients with low grade bladder tumors BECAUSE one can detect recurrences very early in their course.

ANSWERS AND DISCUSSION

1. (C) Gross total painless hematuria is the most common presenting symptom of bladder tumors. It is usually intermittent, and on occasion, it can be terminal hematuria, but is rarely in the initial portion of the stream. The diagnosis is, of course, confirmed by biopsy.

Bladder Tumors

2. (E) Now it is well known that smokers have at least twice the incidence of bladder cancer than do nonsmokers. They have an increased amount of tryptophan metabolites in the urine (similar in chemical structure to 2-naphthylamine) which also have been shown to be etiologic agents in this disease.

3. (C) These are metabolized in the body to ortho-amino-phenols by the liver, conjugated with sulfate and glucuronic acid and excreted in the urine. Then, they are hydrolyzed by the enzyme beta glucuronidase and excreted as ortho-phenols. The latter compounds have been shown to be carcinogenic in laboratory animals.

4. (E) The 5-year survival rate for transitional cell carcinoma, Grade I, is over 75% treated by conservative means as in this case. These are rarely invasive and can go for many years, even in the presence of recurrent tumors.

5. (D) Cytology is not very helpful in low grade malignancy or in papilloma. In higher grade tumors with more anaplasia, it can be very helpful in detecting recurrences, sometimes even before they can be seen cytoscopically.

See Case 43 for references.

CASE 41: 52-YEAR-OLD MALE WITH GROSS HEMATURIA

HISTORY

A 52-year-old male presented with gross total painless hematuria. There was no frequency of urination, dysuria, flank pain, chills, or fever. He had been perfectly well prior to his visit.

PHYSICAL EXAMINATION

Blood pressure: 140-90. Heart and chest were normal. Abdomen was normal. On rectal examination, the prostate was normal and there were no masses palpable on bimanual examination.

LABORATORY DATA

Many RBC per high power field on urinalysis. CBC, urine culture, blood urea nitrogen, FBS, and chest x-ray were all within normal limits. An intravenous urogram showed prompt bilateral excretion with normal upper tracts. Excretory cystogram showed a "cauliflower tumor" (Fig. 41.1). Cystoscopy confirmed the presence of a bladder tumor on the posterior wall of the bladder above the interureteric ridge. It was papillary in nature and on a narrow stalk. Transurethral resection of the lesion was carried out resecting the base of the lesion. Pathologic report was transitional cell carcinoma of the bladder, Grade II, Stage A.

CLINICAL COURSE

Cystoscopy was performed every three months thereafter. Within the year, a second bladder tumor developed, this time on the left lateral wall. This was resected similarly, with the identical pathology found. A third recurrence was noted in six months and again a Grade II, Stage A tumor was resected. He received six instillations of Thio-Tepa following this, and has not had any recurrence of tumor since that time. He has cystoscopy at yearly intervals at present. He has been followed for six years since his original tumor.

QUESTIONS

(T)RUE OR (F)ALSE:

1. Bladder tumors commonly present as cystitis in women.

2. Tumor grade frequently changes with recurrences.

Bladder Tumors

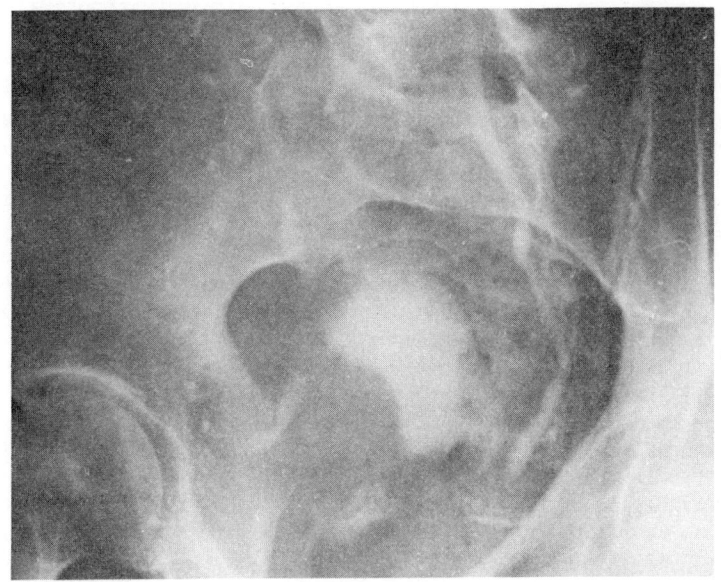

FIG. 41.1: Excretory cystogram showing filling defect in bladder.

3. Well-differentiated bladder tumors are associated with bladder outlet obstruction.

4. Staging of bladder tumors can be accomplished accurately by transurethral resection.

5. Low grade tumors are associated usually with low stages.

MULTIPLE CHOICE:

6. The 5-year survival rate of Grade II, Stage A transitional cell carcinoma treated by transurethral resection can be expected to be:
   A. 20-30%
   B. 30-40%
   C. 45-60%
   D. Over 75%

ANSWERS AND DISCUSSION

1. (T) The marked symptoms of cystitis can be seen as a presenting symptom of bladder tumor. Of course, carcinoma in situ should be considered, and cystoscopic examination would be the differentiating factor here.

2. (F) Tumor grade goes up after recurrences in about 10-15% of cases.

3. (T) In the Bristol Tumor Register, it has been shown that well-differentiated tumors are frequently associated with bladder outlet obstruction.

4. (F) Although transurethral resection is very helpful in staging bladder tumor, it is by no means the most accurate. Every attempt should be made to resect adequate amounts of muscle tissue for adequate histologic examination for invasion. To this must be added bimanual examination, lymphangiography, radioactive isotope studies of liver and bone, as well as other modalities. Surgical exploration for regional lymph node metastases would be the most accurate method of staging. Many patients will be upgraded after this procedure.

5. (T) If a biopsy shows a low grade tumor, there is a 65-75% chance that the stage also will be low. If the tumor is high grade, there is a 75% chance that the stage will be high as well.

6. (C) The 5-year survival rate of this type of tumor treated by TURB alone has ranged from 47% to 57% in one series by Flocks and another by Milner.

See Case 43 for references.

CASE 42: 57-YEAR-OLD MALE WITH GROSS HEMATURIA

HISTORY

A 57-year-old male was admitted to the hospital with gross total painless hematuria of one month's duration. There were no associated urinary symptoms.

He had had a left nephrectomy for stones 30 years ago. He had had a myocardial infarction seven years previously, but made an uneventful recovery and was on no medication for this. He had been a heavy smoker.

PHYSICAL EXAMINATION

Blood pressure: 144/84. Heart and chest were normal. Abdomen was normal with no organs or masses palpable. Bimanual rectal examination showed no evidence of masses.

LABORATORY DATA

Urinalysis revealed many RBCs and 6 to 8 WBCs per high power field. A urine culture showed "a few" colonies of E. coli sensitive to all antibiotics tested. CBC, BUN, FBS, acid, and alkaline phosphatase were all normal.

An intravenous urogram revealed a hypertrophied right kidney, but was otherwise unremarkable. Cystoscopy showed two 2cm papillary lesions on the anterior wall of the bladder, well away from the bladder neck. Several random biopsies of the bladder were normal.

CLINICAL COURSE

Transurethral resection was attempted, but only superficial bites could be obtained, and these revealed fragments of transitional cell carcinoma, Grade II.

Random biopsies from other areas of the bladder were normal. Because removal by transurethral method was unsuccessful, a segmental resection of the bladder was carried out, removing that portion with the two tumors plus a 1" cuff surrounding this area. Two lymph nodes from the area of the hypogastric artery were biopsied and were free of tumor. Pathologic report revealed transitional cell carcinoma, Grade II, Stage B_1 (invasion of superficial muscle).

Postoperatively, the bladder capacity was somewhat small, necessitating frequent voiding, but this gradually increased until an almost normal voiding pattern was obtained. He was cystoscoped at 3-month intervals for one year without evidence of recurrence. He died of a myocardial infarction 14 months after surgery. A postmortem examination could not be obtained.

See Case 43 for questions and references.

Bladder Tumors

CASE 43: 65-YEAR-OLD MALE WITH GROSS HEMATURIA

HISTORY

A 65-year-old male was admitted with a 4-week history of intermittent gross total painless hematuria. There were episodes of nocturia two or three times over the past several years, with some decrease in force and caliber of the urinary stream. Past medical history, review of systems, and family history were essentially negative.

PHYSICAL EXAMINATION

There was a movable mass above the prostate. It was not attached to the pelvic walls. The remainder of the examination was normal.

LABORATORY DATA

All routine studies were normal. Chest x-ray was normal. A cystoscopy revealed a sessile, reddened tumor above and adjacent to the left ureteral orifice. Transurethral resection was performed; superficial and deep portions of the tumor were submitted separately for pathologic analysis. The report revealed infiltrating transitional cell carcinoma, with areas of squamous metaplasia showing deep muscle invasion. In view of the deep extent of the tumor and its close proximity to the ureter, it was elected to perform radical cystectomy. Abdominal exploration was performed. There was no evidence of metastatic disease; radical cystectomy was performed, removing the entire bladder, prostate and seminal vesicles, and all surrounding connective tissue, as well as draining lymph nodes along both hypogastric, external and common iliac chains. An ilial loop diversion was performed. All lymph nodes removed were free of tumor. His postoperative course was benign, except for a prolonged ileus, and he was discharged on the 12th postoperative day. He has been entirely free of symptoms since surgery. Follow-up intravenous urograms are normal. The ileostomy has functioned well without complications. There are no signs of metastatic disease as of the date of this writing.

QUESTIONS: CASES 42-43

1. The 5-year survival rate for a patient with a Grade III, Stage B_2 carcinoma of the bladder treated by segmental resection, can be expected to be:
   A. Less than 10%

B. 10-20%
C. 20-30%
D. 30-40%
E. Over 40%

2. Segmental resection of the bladder for carcinoma should be reserved for patients with:
   A. High grade, low stage tumors
   B. Low grade, low stage tumors
   C. No evidence of metastases
   D. Tumors in the anterior wall and dome
   E. None of the above

3. The expected 5-year survival rate for patients with Grade III or IV, Stage B_2 or C treated by radical cystectomy alone would be:
   A. Less than 10%
   B. 10-20%
   C. 20-30%
   D. 30-40%
   E. Over 40%

4. The expected 5-year survival rate for patients with Grade III or IV, Stage B_2 or C treated by preoperative radiotherapy and radical cystectomy would be:
   A. Less than 10%
   B. 10-20%
   C. 20-30%
   D. 30-40%
   E. 40-50%

5. Which of the following may be of value in the diagnosis of carcinoma of the bladder?
   A. Hg^{203}
   B. Fuidan
   C. Tetracycline
   D. Atabrine
   E. None of the above

6. The natural history of a significant number of bladder carcinoma in situ is:
   A. Static
   B. Progressive to infiltration
   C. Eventual disappearance
   D. Not known
   E. Very variable

Bladder Tumors

ANSWERS AND DISCUSSION: CASES 42-43

1. (E) Utz, et al., in a review of 199 patients at the Mayo Clinic, treated by Segmental Resection only, found that the 5-year survival rate for Stage B_2 tumors was 40%, and was 29% for Stage C. Forty-seven percent of patients with Grade III tumors survived five years and 21% of patients with Grade IV survived that long. There have been even higher figures reported in the literature, but not in as great numbers as this series.

2. (D) The problem with Segmental Resection for bladder tumor is in proper selection. Grade and stage of the tumor really should not enter the decision. The tumor must be in an area of the bladder where a good margin of the bladder which is free of tumor can be resected. Of course, there must be no metastases present. One must be absolutely certain that there are no changes in other parts of the bladder indicating that tumors may form there, such as atypia or carcinoma in situ. This is confirmed by random cup biopsies, as in Case 42. We now would use preoperative radiotherapy in this situation.

3. (B) Preoperative radiotherapy combined with radical
4. (E) cystectomy has been clearly shown to be better than either modality used alone. This would be reserved for patients with Stages B_2 and C, or possibly D_1, since more conservative forms of therapy would suffice for less invasive tumors. Most series of patients treated with preoperative radiotherapy and cystectomy report 5-year survival rates of 40-50%. Research is continuing vigorously in this field.

5. (C) Tetracycline, when administered, causes fluorescence of neoplastic areas of the bladder when examined under ultraviolet light cystoscopically. Suspicious areas may fluoresce even though no gross tumor is seen. These then can be biopsied.

6. (B) In a series of 62 patients, Utz found that 82% had recurrence after treatment and deterioration in grade 52%; 73% of these patients showing infiltration.

REFERENCES: CASES 40-43

1. Uroepithelial tumors. Urol Clin N Amer, Vol. 3, No. 1, Feb. 1976.

2. Russell Scott, Jr. (ed.), Controversies in Urology, Chapter 3, W.B. Saunders Company, Philadelphia, 1972, p. 51.

3. Utz DC, et al.: A clinicopathologic evaluation of partial cystectomy for carcinoma of the bladder. Cancer 32:1075, Nov. 1973.

4. Utz DC, et al.: In situ carcinoma of the bladder. J Urol 103:162, 1970.

5. Whitmore WF, Jr: The treatment of bladder tumors. Surg Clin N Amer 49:349, 1969.

CHAPTER VIII

CARCINOMA OF THE PROSTATE

INTRODUCTION

Carcinoma of the prostate is the most common cancer of the genitourinary tract in men and the second most common cancer seen in all men. The incidence has been said to be 25% in men past the age of 70. Unfortunately, the diagnosis usually is made late in the course of the disease because there is lack of symptoms until the disease has spread to local surrounding structures and has metastasized to regional lymph nodes, bone, liver, brain, etc.

The etiology of prostatic carcinoma is unknown, although its dependence on hormones is well known. Androgens are known to increase the rate of growth of the tumor. Estrogen therapy or orchiectomy slows their growth and will decrease the level of acid phosphatase mediated by the prostate.

The lesion usually starts in the posterior lobe of the gland adjacent to the rectum and can be diagnosed easily by palpation in the early stages prior to development of symptoms. It gradually spreads locally and involves the entire prostate, urethra, bladder base; it spreads by venous as well as lymphatic channels. Rarely does it involve the rectum. The microscopic picture is either scirrhous or adenocarcinomatous. In the scirrhous type, columns of darkly stained cells infiltrate the gland and are separated by a fibrous stroma. In the adenocarcinomatous type, the cells are large and have an irregular acinar formation. The basement membrane is lost. Generally, the more well-differentiated tumors respond best to hormone therapy.

Treatment can be divided into four (4) modes of therapy: a) hormonal; b) surgical; c) radiotherapy; and d) chemotherapy. Hormonal can be by use of various synthetic estrogens (Tace®, diethylstilbestrol). Recently, the use of various antiandrogen progestational agents have been shown to be effective in the treatment of advanced carcinoma of the prostate. Bilateral orchiectomy can be performed at the time of diagnosis, or when metastases develop. Radical surgery is reserved for those clinically manifest tumors that are confined to the prostate and show no signs of local spread or metastases. This involves removal of the prostate, seminal vesicles, and surrounding fascia. The bladder neck is anastomosed to the membranous urethra. It may be performed via the retropubic or perineal route. Palliative surgery generally is performed for the relief of symptoms of urinary obstruction. Transurethral resection of the obstructing tissue is the method of choice.

The use of local infiltration of radioactive iodine into the prostatic tumor with node dissection has been advocated by Whitmore with good results. External radiation using cobalt has been shown to be very beneficial in patients with extensive local disease, and is becoming more popular. Both do not carry with them the relatively high morbidity rate of incontinence and impotence seen after radical prostatectomy.

Carcinoma of the Prostate

CASE 44: 62-YEAR-OLD MALE WITH DIFFICULTY VOIDING

HISTORY

A 62-year-old male was seen for increasing symptoms of prostatism. He had nocturia 2-3 times, decrease in force and caliber of his urinary stream, and straining to urinate. He denied hematuria, dysuria, frequency or urgency of urination. He had had a myocardial infarction five years previously, but as far as his heart was concerned, has been asymptomatic.

PHYSICAL EXAMINATION

Blood pressure: 120/74. Heart and chest negative. Abdomen negative. Genitalia normal. The prostate was smooth and felt benign and was approximately 25 to 30mg in size.

LABORATORY DATA

Urinalysis normal. CBC normal. Blood urea nitrogen 17mg%. Creatinine 0.7mg%. An intravenous urogram showed normal upper tracts. There was a residual urine on the postvoid film of approximately 90cc of urine. Cystopanendoscopy revealed a trabeculated bladder and an obstructing prostate gland.

CLINICAL COURSE

The patient underwent transurethral resection of the prostate, and 25 grams of tissue were removed. He made an uneventful postoperative recovery. Pathologic examination of the specimen revealed a focus of adenocarcinoma within a benign enlargement of the gland. Numerous sections then were taken and examined, but no other focus of carcinoma was seen. No further therapy was given. The patient has been observed for five years and seven months without any further evidence of tumor.

QUESTIONS

1. Into which clinical stage of prostate carcinoma would this patient be classified?
    A. Stage O
    B. Stage A_1
    C. Stage A_2
    D. Stage B_1
    E. Stage B_2

2. What percentage of patients with carcinoma of the prostate found only on microscopic section will progress to metastases?
   A. 2%
   B. 5-10%
   C. 11-20%
   D. 30%

3. The proper therapy for diffuse microscopic involvement of an otherwise apparently benign gland would be:
   A. Observation only
   B. Radical prostatectomy
   C. Megavoltage radiotherapy
   D. Bilateral orchiectomy
   E. B or C

ANSWERS AND DISCUSSION

1. (B) Carcinoma of the prostate, without metastases and apparently only on microscopic section, is classified Stage A. These have been classified further into Stage A_1 and Stage A_2. The former comprise the majority of these tumors and are truly microsopic and have a low biologic potential. A small percentage of Stage A tumors will have a larger volume and be more diffusely invasive within the gland, and will generally be of a higher grade of malignancy. They are classified Stage A_2. These generally are more aggressive and require further therapy either by radical excision or megavoltage radiotherapy.

2. (B) The Veterans Administration Cooperative Study found 262 cases of Stage A cancer. Death from tumor occurred in only five patients (1.9%). Only 6.8% of these patients showed any evidence of advancing cancer.

3. (E) Evidence of diffuse microscopic involvement or high grade of tumor in Stage A would require further therapy of some type. This would be either in the form of radical excision or megavoltage radiotherapy. Bilateral orchiectomy generally would be reserved for those patients with symptomatic metastatic disease.

REFERENCE

1. Byar DR and Veterans Administration Cooperative Urologic Group: Survival of patients with incidentally found microscopic cancer of the prostate: Results of a clinical trial of conservative treatment. J Urol 108:908, 1972.

Carcinoma of the Prostate

CASE 45: 58-YEAR-OLD MALE WITH FREQUENCY

HISTORY

A 58-year-old male was referred to the urologist because of frequency every 2 hours during the day and nocturia 2 to 3 times. He complained of hesitancy and decrease in force and caliber of his urinary stream over the past several years. He denied hematuria. He had had a myocardial infarction in 1957 and had made a complete recovery, his ECG returning to normal. In 1963, he had a left ureteral colic and passed a small calculus. There was a history of primary syphilis 25 years before, with a negative serology subsequently. Review of systems was otherwise negative.

PHYSICAL EXAMINATION

Positive findings were limited to the rectal examination. The prostate was 1+ to 2+ enlarged. On the right side, near the base, was a small, firm nodule which was less than 1.0cm in diameter. It was smooth but definitely harder than the remainder of the gland.

LABORATORY DATA

All routine checks were normal. A Vim-Silverman needle biopsy of the prostate was performed and revealed adenocarcinoma. Metastatic bone survey and phosphatase, and posterior iliac crest bone marrow biopsy were all negative for metastatic disease.

CLINICAL COURSE

A radical retropubic prostatectomy and lymphadenectomy was performed removing the entire prostate and seminal vesicles. All lymph nodes were negative. Postoperative course was uneventful and the catheter was removed on the 13th postoperative day. He voided with a good stream but poor control. By the 18th postoperative day, he had regained complete diurnal control, but had some enuresis which disappeared gradually. He has remained asymptomatic with no evidence of metastases to date.

QUESTIONS

1. In patients with Stage B carcinoma of the prostate (confined to the gland), regional lymph nodes may be involved in:
    A. Less than 10% of cases
    B. 10-20% of cases

Case 45 / Carcinoma of the Prostate

C. 20-30% of cases
D. 30-40% of cases
E. More than 40% of cases

2. The initial lymph nodes involved in carcinoma of the prostate are generally:
    A. Hypogastric
    B. External iliac
    C. Common iliac
    D. Obturator

3. The indications for radical prostatectomy are:
    A. Discrete nodule (1cm or less)
    B. Compressible tissue on two sides
    C. No fixation of the prostate
    D. No evidence of metastases
    E. All of the above

4. An advantage of radical retropubic prostatectomy is:
    A. Decreased incontinence
    B. Decreased impotence
    C. Visualization of regional lymph nodes
    D. Less blood loss
    E. None of the above

5. After radical prostatectomy, the expected 15-year survivial rate would be:
    A. Less than 10%
    B. 10-20%
    C. 20-30%
    D. 30-40%
    E. Over 40%

ANSWERS AND DISCUSSION

1. (C) It has been shown by Flocks and others that the incidence of lymph node metastases increases with increase in size of the lesion. An incidence of approximately 25% of patients with tumor apparently confined to the gland, will show evidence of lymph node metastases.

2. (D) The earliest lymph node involvement generally is the obturator nodes on the side of the lesion.

3. (E) For radical prostatectomy to be done, the patient must have a discrete, preferably small nodule in the prostate, with compressible tissue on at least two sides of it. There

Carcinoma of the Prostate

must be no fixation of the gland or induration of the seminal vesicles. There must be no clinical laboratory or x-ray evidence of metastases. The patient must be in good general health and preferably not more than 70 years of age.

4. (C) Radical retropubic prostatectomy allows regional lymph node dissection and accurate staging of the disease. We do this prior to performing the prostatectomy and submit excised nodes for frozen section. If the nodes are involved, the procedure is abandoned. The incidence of impotence, incontinence and blood loss is about equal to that of radical perineal prostatectomy.

5. (D) Jewett, who has probably the largest personal experience with radical perineal prostatectomy, has a 33%, 15-year survival rate.

See Case 46 for references.

CASE 46: 66-YEAR-OLD MALE WITH NODULE OF PROSTATE

HISTORY

A 66-year-old male was referred because of a nodule found by his internist on routine physical examination. He had mild symptoms of hesitancy of his urinary stream and only occasional nocturia. He denied hematuria or other urinary symptoms. His only significant past history was a left inguinal hernia repair.

PHYSICAL EXAMINATION

Blood pressure 160/110. There was a firm nodule palpable on the right side of the prostate that apparently was confined to the gland. There was no fixation of the prostate. The mass was approximately 1-2cm in diameter. The remainder of the examination was normal.

LABORATORY DATA

Urinalysis and CBC normal. BUN and creatinine normal. Chest x-ray normal. Liver and bone scan normal. Acid phosphatase normal. Bone marrow normal with no evidence of tumor. Intravenous urogram showed normal upper tracts. There was only a small residual urine.

CLINICAL COURSE

A needle biopsy of the prostate revealed well-differentiated adenocarcinoma. The diagnosis and further management were discussed in detail with the patient. It was elected to treat him with super voltage x-ray therapy. He has been followed for 6 years postoperatively and he is doing well. He is asymptomatic, and there is no evidence of metastases.

QUESTIONS

1. Clinical Stage B prostatic cancer will show nodal metastases in:
   A. Less than 10%
   B. 10-35%
   C. 40-55%
   D. 55-60%
   E. More than 65%

2. The initial site of nodal metastases in prostatic carcinoma is:

Carcinoma of the Prostate Case 46/ 221

    A. External iliac nodes
    B. Inguinal lymph nodes
    C. Obturator nodes
    D. Presacral nodes
    E. Common iliac nodes

3. Bipedal lymphangiography will be accurate in detecting normal metastases in:
    A. No cases
    B. 10% of cases
    C. 50% of cases
    D. 70% of cases
    E. 90% of cases

4. The most reliable method of obtaining specimens of suspected prostatic carcinoma is:
    A. Needle biopsy
    B. Transurethral prostatic resection
    C. Open perineal biopsy
    D. Transrectal biopsy
    E. Enucleation suprapubic prostatectomy

5. Carcinoma will be found in serial sections of the prostate gland in what percent of men over 50?
    A. 5-10%
    B. 15-20%
    C. 25-30%
    D. 35-40%
    E. 45-50%

6. The 10-year survival rate of patients with Stage B carcinoma of the prostate treated by megavoltage radiotherapy is:
    A. Less than 10%
    B. 10-20%
    C. 20-30%
    D. 30-40%
    E. 40-50%

7. The 10-year survival rate of patients with Stage C carcinoma of the prostate treated by megavoltage radiotherapy is:
    A. Less than 10%
    B. 10-20%
    C. 20-30%
    D. 30-40%
    E. 40-50%

8. The 10-year survival rate of patients with Stage B carcinoma of the prostate treated by radical prostatectomy is:
   A. Less than 10%
   B. 10-20%
   C. 20-30%
   D. 30-40%
   E. 40-50%

ANSWERS AND DISCUSSION

1. (B) In the Memorial Hospital Series[1] in which pelvic lymph node dissection was performed for staging, 6 of 29 patients (21%) with Stage B disease had positive nodes. In Stage C disease, 20 of 31 patients (65%) had positive nodes.

2. (C) In the above series, the obturator nodes were involved in 35% of all patients; the external iliac nodes in 23%. The internal iliac (hypogastric) and the common iliac lymph nodes were involved in only 8% and 7%, respectively.

3. (E) In the same series, the accuracy in both Stages B and C was 91%. There was better correlation in Stage C (100%) than Stage B (87%).

4. (C) Needle biopsy of the prostate can often miss the suspected nodule, since it is essentially a blind biopsy. In open perineal biopsy, the nodule actually can be seen as well as palpated and biopsied accurately. TUR biopsy and enucleation specimens are the least accurate.

5. (B) The incidence of carcinoma of the prostate will increase progressively each decade beyond 50, and the overall incidence over 50 is 17%.

6. (E) In Bagshaw's Series treated by external radiotherapy, the 10-year survival rate for Stage B disease was 45%, for Stage C disease, it was 31%.

7. (D)

8. (E) In Jewett's Series of radical prostatectomy, the 10-year survival rate was 52%.

REFERENCES: CASES 45-46

1. Hilaris BS, et al.: Radiation therapy and pelvic node dissection in the management of cancer of the prostate. Am J of Roentgen 121:324, 1974.

2. Pistenma DA, Ray ER, and Bagshaw MA: The role of megavoltage radiation therapy in the treatment of prostate carcinoma. Seminars in Oncology 3, No. 2, June, 1976.

3. Jewett HJ: The present status of radical prostatectomy for Stages A and B prostatic cancer. Urol Clin N Amer 2, No. 1, February 1975.

CHAPTER IX

RENAL CALCULI

INTRODUCTION

The presence of calculi in the urinary tract is termed urolithiasis. A stone can be present in a calyx, pelvis of the kidney, ureter, bladder, bladder diverticulum, urethra, or prostate. The occurrence of stones in the aforementioned areas was known to the ancients. Vesical calculi have been found in Egyptian mummies dating back 7,000 years, and a renal calculus was found in one mummy thought to be 4,000 years old.

There are many factors in stone formation. It is often impossible to identify the cause of an individual calculus. Rarely is one factor alone responsible. Accordingly, a foolproof method of prevention is not known. Calculi vary in their chemical composition and, therefore, in their x-ray appearance. Uric acid and xanthine stones are radiolucent. Calcium, cystine, and mixed stones are radiopaque. At least 90% of calculi contain calcium or magnesium in combination with phosphate or oxalate. The remainder are of organic composition (cystine, uric acid).

One cause of recurrent nephrolithiasis is hyperparathyroidism. Elevated serum calcium is the screening procedure for this malady. Daily serum calciums and phosphorus are taken, as well as 24-hour urinary calcium. Although bone disease is unusual in primary hyperparathyroidism today, examination of the teeth for absence of the lamina dura, as well as x-ray of the hand for subperiosteal resorption of the phalanges should be taken. Should there be evidence of hyperparathyroidism, then parathyroidectomy should be carried out prior to removal of the calculus.

Idiopathic hypercalciuria is probably a more common etiologic factor in stone formation, and is diagnosed by the excretion of more than 180mg of calcium in the urine in 24 hours. One usually leaves the patient on a normal diet for this determination and, if this is elevated, it is repeated on a low calcium intake. Treatment of this condition has been aimed at decreasing the calcium excretion by altered diet, administration of acid phosphate and, lately, by the administration of magnesium oxide.

Urinary stasis and infection are two important factors in urinary lithiasis that must be ruled out. Stasis encourages stone formation by allowing sedimentation of crystals and gravel. Infection can raise the pH of the urine, primarily in the presence of urea-splitting organisms such as Proteus and Pseudomonas. A pH above 7 generally is obtained; and, at this high level, triple phosphate and calcium carbonate are deposited.

Other causes of increased calcium excretion include prolonged immobilization, hypervitaminosis D, excessive milk intake and renal tubular acidosis. All these must be ruled out in the patient with hypercalciuria.

Uric acid stones account for approximately 10% of all renal calculi seen in this country. They generally are caused by excessive tissue breakdown. These calculi are radiolucent and, at times, can be extremely difficult to diagnose. They form in an acid urine, and alkalinization of the urine is important therapy in their prevention. Allopurinol and alkalinization of the urine have been reported to dissolve uric acid calculi.

Cystine stones are a variety of renal calculi, forming in patients with cystinuria, a rare hereditary disease. The latter is due to a defect in renal tubular reabsorption of the amino acids ornithine, lysine, arginine, as well as cystine.

CASE 47: 39-YEAR-OLD MALE WITH PAINLESS HEMATURIA

HISTORY

A 39-year-old male presented with an episode of painless gross hematuria devoid of clots.

LABORATORY DATA

An excretory urogram was performed, but there was no evidence of obstruction, filling defects or radiopacities in the course of the urinary tract.

Cystoscopy revealed no bladder tumor. Thereafter, on numerous occasions, red blood cells were found in the routine urinalysis.

CLINICAL COURSE

He had another episode of gross hematuria, and 4 months later, the above studies were repeated. A radiopacity of 1.2 x 0.75cm was noted in the region of the right renal pelvis (Fig. 47.1), and was confirmed by excretory urography (Fig. 47.2).

The patient was admitted to the hospital, where serum calcium, phosphorus, alkaline phosphatase, and uric acid were normal on 5 occasions. A 24-hour urinary calcium excretion was 100mg, within the normal range. A right pyelolithotomy was performed.

The patient made an uneventful recovery. The stone was composed of calcium oxalate. He has not had a recurrence in 5 years.

See Case 48 for Questions.

Renal Calculi

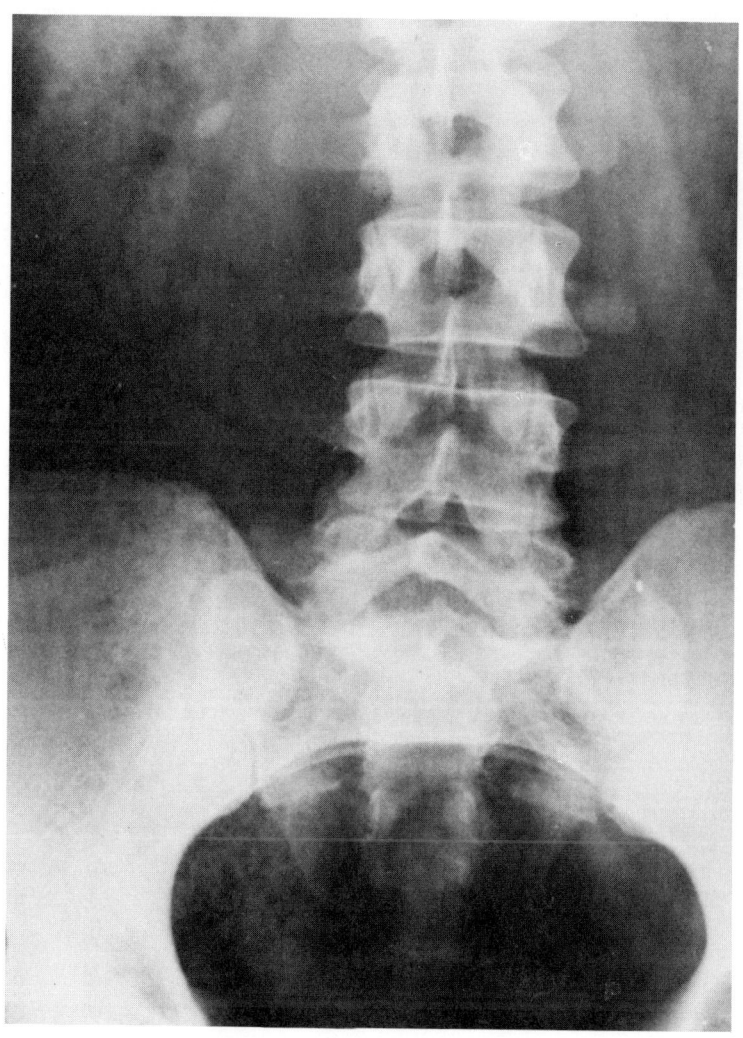

FIG. 47.1: Radiopacity seen in area of right renal pelvis.

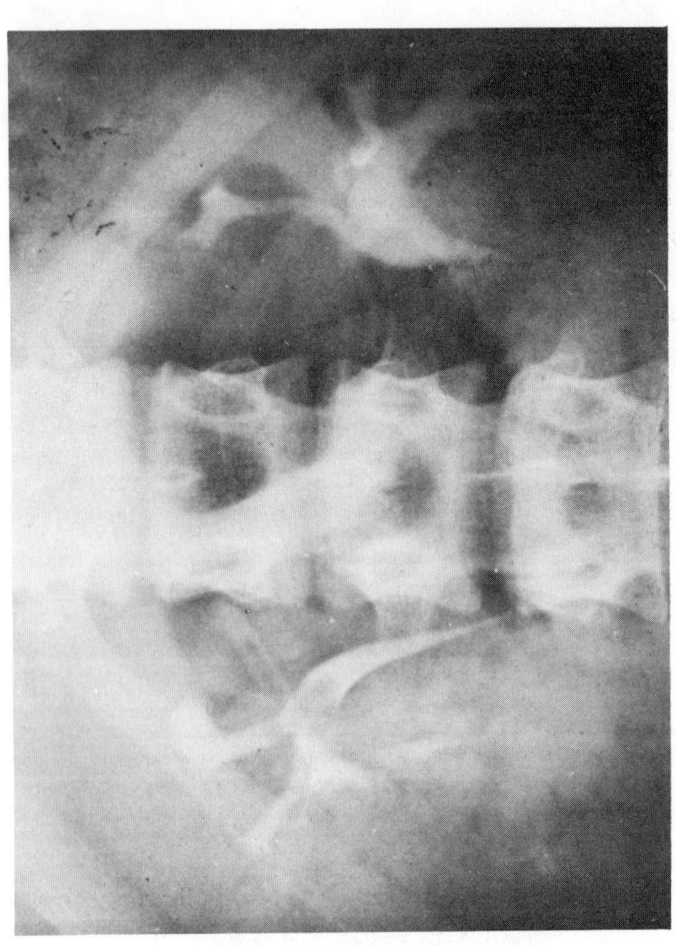

FIG. 47.2: Excretory urography in same patient as Fig. 47.1. Note filling defect in right renal pelvis.

Renal Calculi

CASE 48: 41-YEAR-OLD MALE WITH RENAL COLIC

HISTORY

A 41-year-old male presented with typical right renal colic.

PHYSICAL EXAMINATION

Negative, except for mild right costovertebral angle tenderness.

LABORATORY DATA

Urinalysis was negative. A plain film of the abdomen demonstrated numerous radiopaque shadows in the bony pelvis. An excretory urogram was performed, and delayed opacification of the right collecting system was noted. At 35 minutes, a right hydroureter with columnization to the right ureterovesical junction where the offending calculus was located, was demonstrable (Fig. 48.1).

CLINICAL COURSE

The patient was treated conservatively, and passed the calculus in 9 days. Serum calcium, phosphorus and uric acid determinations were all normal. Twenty-four hour urinary calcium excretion was normal. The stone consisted of calcium oxalate.

Two years and 5 months later, the patient returned with a left renal colic, and a plain film demonstrated a 1.0cm irregular calculus at the interval between the second and third lumbar vertebrae (Fig. 48.2). He was in severe pain, unrelieved by narcotics. Excretory urogram demonstrated a nephrogram in 5 minutes, and a right hydroureteronephrosis down to the level of the offending calculus on the 3-minute film (Fig. 48.3). The patient was observed in the hospital for 4 days, and remained in pain almost constantly. He underwent a left ureterolithotomy. The postoperative course was uneventful. Since that time, he has passed one calculus.

QUESTIONS: CASES 47-48

1. The most common type of renal calculi is:
    A. Uric acid
    B. Magnesium ammonium phosphate
    C. Calcium carbonate
    D. Calcium oxalate
    E. Phosphate stone

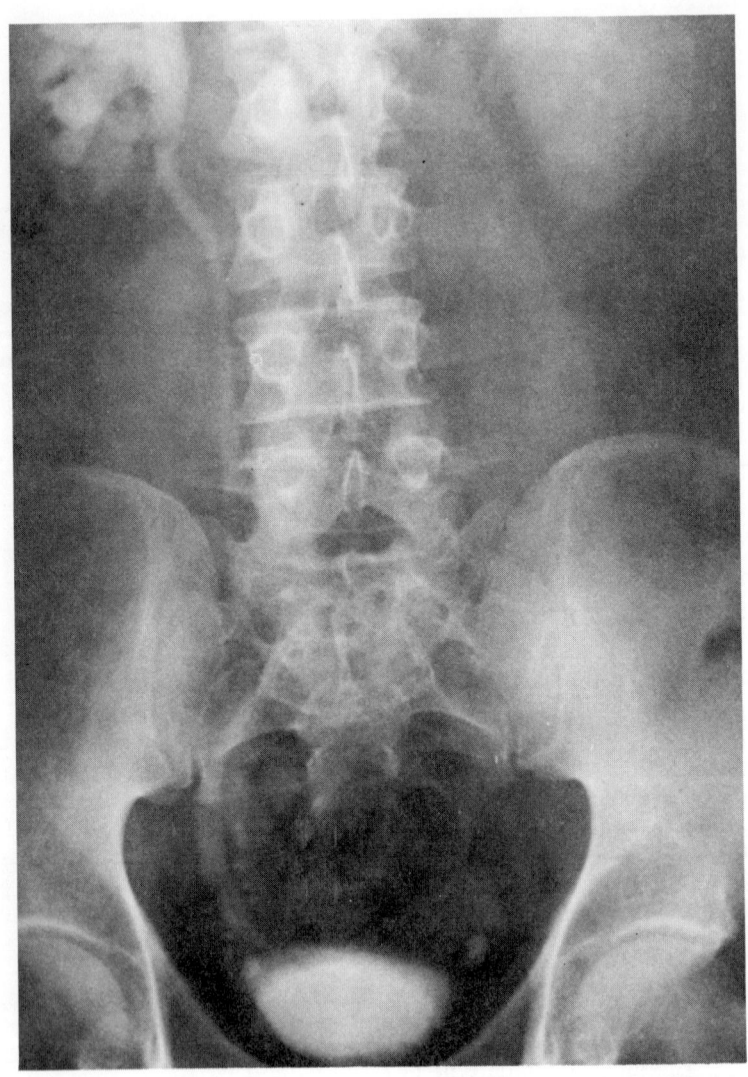

FIG. 48.1: A 35-minute excretory urogram showing columnization to the right ureterovesical junction.

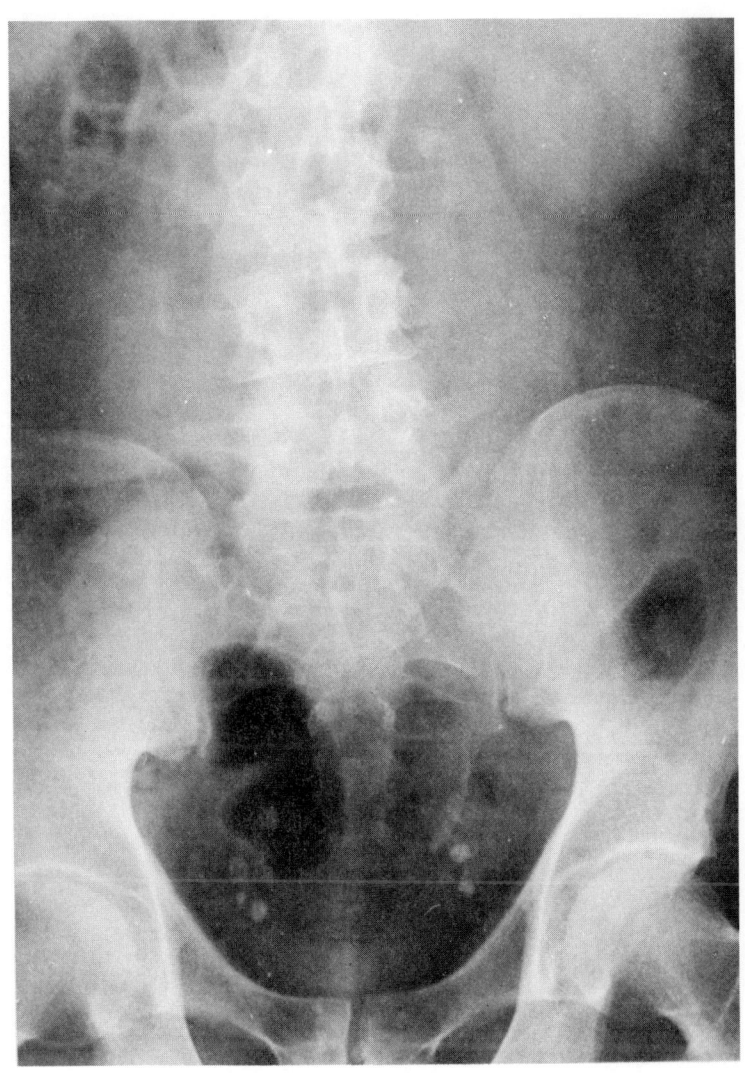

FIG. 48.2: A 1.0cm calculus is seen at L2 - L3.

232/ Case 48   Renal Calculi

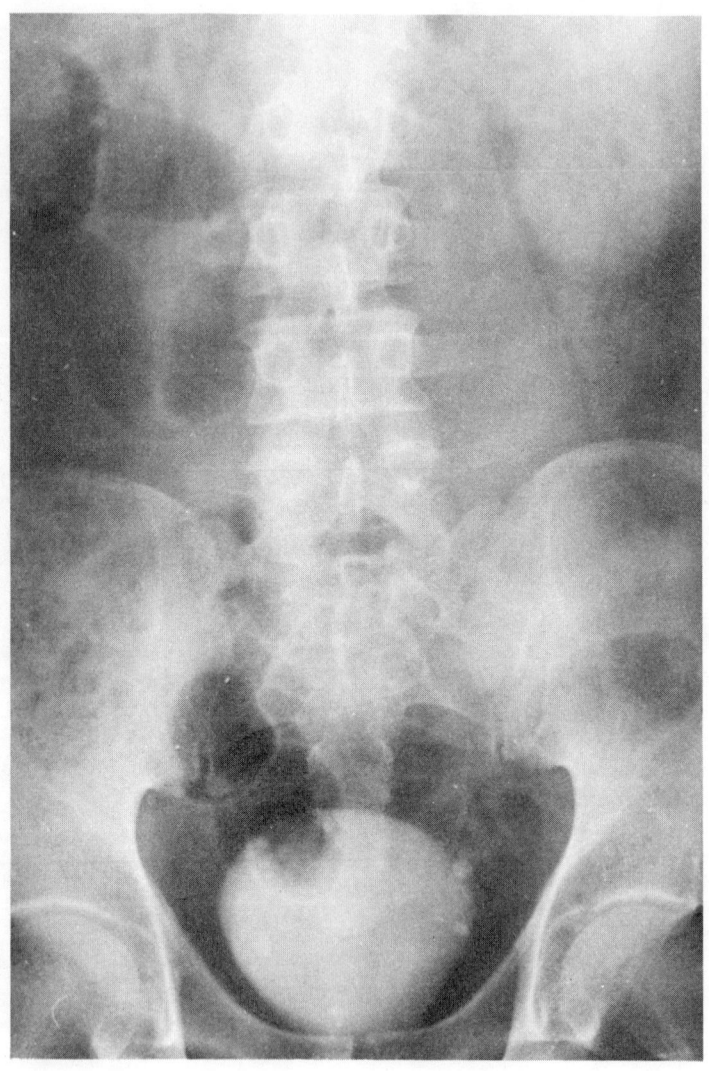

FIG. 48.3: Left hydroureteronephrosis down to the offending calculus.

Renal Calculi

2. The most common site of calculus production in the urinary tract is:
   A. The bladder
   B. The urethra
   C. The ureter
   D. The kidney
   E. The renal pelvis

3. An intravenous urogram which opacifies the entire renal parenchyma without visualizing the collecting system is indicative of:
   A. Renal artery occlusion
   B. Renal vein occlusion
   C. Intrarenal hemorrhage
   D. Ureteral obstruction

MATCH THE FOLLOWING NORMAL VALUES WITH THE APPROPRIATE CHEMICAL IN A 24-HOUR EXCRETION OF URINE:

4. ___ Cystine   A. 0.06-0.2gm
5. ___ Oxalate   B. 2.5-3.5gm
6. ___ Calcium   C. 0.01-0.03gm
7. ___ Uric acid   D. 0.4-1.0gm
8. ___ Phosphate   E. Trace

MATCH THE FOLLOWING:

9. ___ Hereditary defect   A. Calcium oxalate
10. ___ Infectious concretions   B. Magnesium ammonium
11. ___ Radiolucent
12. ___ Nephrocalcinosis   C. Cystine
13. ___ "Ground glass" appearance   D. Uric acid
    on x-ray

14. Indications for surgery in ureteral calculus would include all of the following except:
    A. Unremitting pain
    B. Hydronephrosis
    C. Fever of 102°
    D. Gross hematuria
    E. Calculus greater than 5mm

ANSWERS AND DISCUSSION: CASES 47-48

1. (D) The majority of calculi in the United States are of calcium oxalate. Calculi that occur in an apparently normal urinary tract with an acid urine generally are calcium oxalate,

or a mixture of calcium oxalate and calcium phosphate. Magnesium ammonium phosphate stones occur in an alkaline urine, and generally are associated with urea-splitting organisms.

Uric acid stones comprise about 8-10% of all stones seen, and cystine stones comprise less than 1-2% of those seen.

2. (D) In the United States, the most common site of stone formation in the urinary tract is within the kidney. The initial event causing stone formation remains controversial and obscure, but numerous factors probably play a role. All agree that some nidus for precipitation of crystalloid material is the initiating factor. Whether this is organic matrix or crystalloid in nature remains unsolved.

3. (D) A nephrogram is indicative of acute ureteral occlusion, and represents concentration of the contrast material within the tubules of the kidney. The occluded ureter and hydronephrotic collecting system, with its increased pressure, prevent excretion of the substance into the collecting system.

4. (E)
5. (C)
6. (A)
7. (D)
8. (B)

The normal 24-hour values for these substances are shown. The excretion of the substances are important to determine, in order to establish an etiology for stone formation, as well as establish appropriate treatment. Hypercalciuria can be secondary to hypercalcemia, or be dietary or renal in origin. This would be essential to determine, in order to treat this condition. More than trace amounts of cystine in a 24-hour urine should alert one to the possibility of this being an etiology of stone formation, and appropriate medical management should be given. Hyperoxaluria is a rare cause of stone formation.

9. (C)
10. (B)
11. (D)
12. (A)
13. (C)

Cystinuria is a familial disease, being inherited as a recessive or incompletely recessive trait. It is one of the least soluble of the amino acids and, when excreted in large amounts, is saturated and easily precipitated. It has the typical "ground glass" appearance on x-ray. As stated previously, magnesium phosphate stones generally are associated with infections of urea-splitting organisms. Uric acid stones are radiolucent and, characteristically, are seen only as filling defects on intravenous urography.

Calcific deposits within the renal parenchyma in nephrocalcinosis are invariably composed of calcium oxalate.

14. (D) Gross hematuria with ureteral calculi rarely is sufficient to require surgical intervention. The other criteria listed are those used as indications for surgery.

CASE 49: 65-YEAR-OLD FEMALE WITH HEMATURIA

HISTORY

A 65-year-old female presented a history of hematuria of three days' duration. She stated that her right kidney had been removed 10 years previously but could not say why. She had been in perfect health since that time.

PHYSICAL EXAMINATION

The blood pressure was 220/100. Heart and chest were normal. Abdomen soft and flat. There was no CVA tenderness.

LABORATORY DATA

Included a urinalysis which showed innumerable RBCs and 2+ protein. Blood urea nitrogen 21mg%, uric acid 9.7mg%, glucose 177mg%. Hemoglobin 12.5gm%. A drip infusion I.V. urogram showed prompt excretion on the left with good visualization of the collecting system, as well as the entire left ureter. In the left renal pelvis was a large translucent area suggestive of a nonopaque calculus measuring approximately 3.0cm in length. This was confirmed by films taken in the oblique, PA, PA and prone view (Fig. 49.1).

CLINICAL COURSE

A left pyelolithotomy was performed and a calculus measuring 2.8 x 2.2 x 0.9cm was removed from the renal pelvis. Chemical analysis was uric acid. Patient made an uneventful recovery. She was placed on Allopurinol and sodium bicarbonate and advised to titrate her urine with pH paper, with which she has done quite well. A repeat excretory urogram showed a normal left collecting system. She has not had a recurrence of stone for the past seven years, and her renal function remains normal.

QUESTIONS

1. The incidence of renal lithiasis in gouty patients is:
    A. Less than 5%
    B. 10-30%
    C. 40-50%
    D. 75%

2. The mechanism of action of allopurinol primarily:
    A. Increases urinary pH

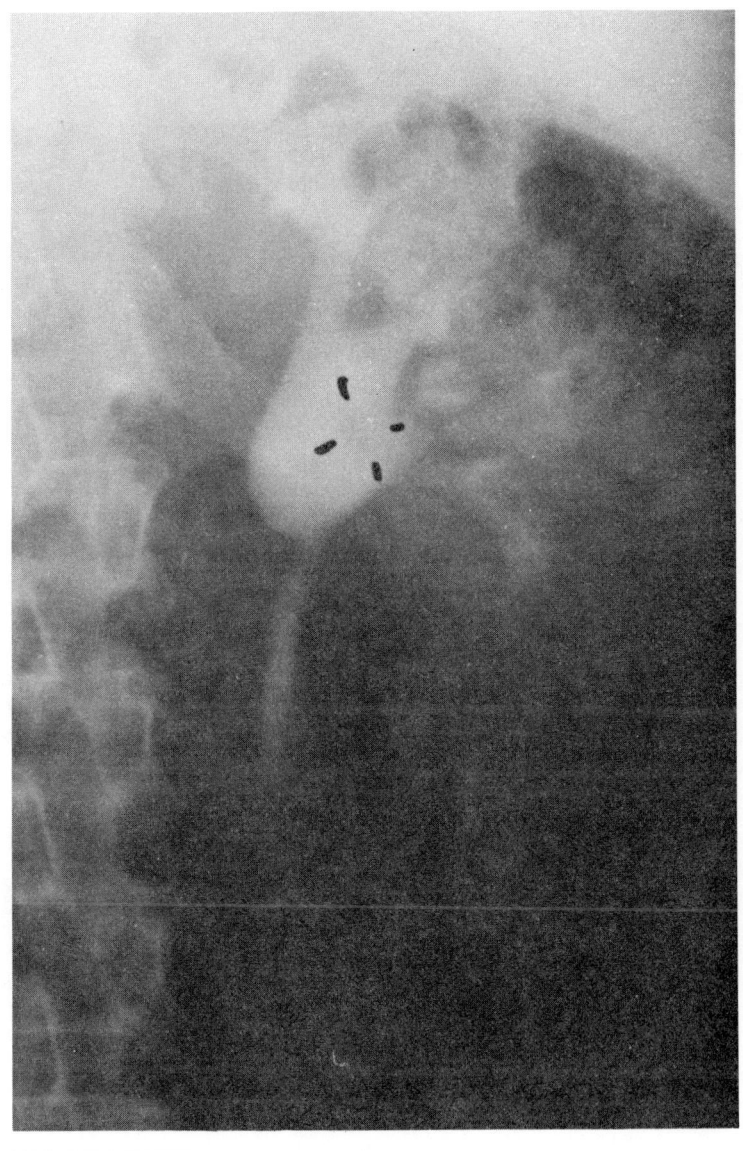

FIG. 49.1: Intravenous urogram showing filling defect in the left renal pelvis consistent with uric acid calculus.

B. Decreases uric acid excretion
C. Decreases uric acid production
D. Increases solubility or uric acid

3. Hyperuricemia in gout is secondary to:
   A. Low excretion of uric acid by the kidneys
   B. Increased xanthine oxidase enzymatic action
   C. Lack of xanthine oxidase enzymatic action
   D. Increased hypoxanthine oxidase enzymatic action

EACH OF THE FOLLOWING STATEMENTS CONSISTS OF A STATEMENT AND A REASON. ANSWER BY USING THE FOLLOWING KEY:

A. If both statement and reason are true and related cause and effect
B. If both statement and reason are true but not related cause and effect
C. If the statement is true, but the reason false
D. If the statement is false, but the reason true
E. If both statement and reason are false

4. A negative x-ray film does not rule out urinary calculi BECAUSE a pneumopyelogram may cause the calculus to stand out sharply.

5. Renal stones which are over one centimeter and are free in the pelvis demand surgical treatment BECAUSE the danger of the stone in the kidney generally is much greater than that of surgical intervention.

6. In considering renal surgery, the size of the calculus, rather than the site, is the most important consideration BECAUSE large stones are removed more easily.

ANSWERS AND DISCUSSION

1. (B) The incidence of renal lithiasis in gouty patients ranges from 5-30%, depending on the series consulted. With rising levels of serum uric acid, the incidence of calculi also increases. In Israel, the incidence of calculus disease in gouty patients is 75% and may be secondary to the hot climate, as well as genetic factors.

2. (C) Allopurinol blocks the action of xanthine oxidase, thus blocking the formation of uric acid in the body. Increased amounts of xanthine are therefore formed and excreted. The incidence of xanthine stones is extremely rare.

Renal Calculi   Case 49/ 239

3. (B) The error is metabolism of purine in patients with gout results from increased action of the enzyme xanthine oxidase. Hypoxanthine and xanthine then are converted into an excessive amount of uric acid which is then presented to the kidneys and excreted in increased amounts. This causes an increased concentration in uric acid in the urine; coupled with a tendency toward hyperacidity in the urine in these patients, uric acid stones form.

4. (B) Both statements are true but the reason does not relate to the statement. Air pyelograms frequently are useful in outlining filling defects of question in intravenous urography. However, they will not differentiate tumor from stone. If the stone is large enough, sonography may be helpful.

5. (B) Stones larger than 1cm rarely will pass if they do go into the ureter; invariably they are obstructive and require surgical intervention.

6. (E) Both statements are false.

CASE 50: 52-YEAR-OLD FEMALE WITH HEMATURIA AND FLANK PAIN

HISTORY

A 52-year-old female was seen initially in November, 1977 because of gross hematuria and mild right flank pain. There were no chills nor fever. Twenty years previously, she had a left nephrectomy for calculous disease. She was a heroin addict for many years and was on Methadone maintenance for the past two years. A plain film of abdomen in November, 1977 showed no evidence of calculi. An intravenous urogram showed caliectasis and cupping of the lower calyces on the right, indicative of probable papillary necrosis (Figs. 50.1 and 50.2). Cystoscopy at this time was negative, and she was discharged to have a repeat excretory urogram in three months.

She was totally asymptomatic until early February, 1978 when she presented to the emergency room stating that she had not voided in the past 36 hours. She also complained of some right flank pain, as well as chills and fever. She was admitted immediately.

PHYSICAL EXAMINATION

BP 140/80. Temperature 100.4°. Respiration 18. There was marked right upper quadrant and right CVA tenderness. She was alert and lucid. The remainder of the physical examination was within normal limits.

LABORATORY DATA

Hemoglobin 12.5gm%, hematocrit 39%, blood urea nitrogen 61 mg%, creatinine 3.2mg%. Blood urea nitrogen and creatinine had been normal three months previously. Chemical profile was otherwise within normal limits.

CLINICAL COURSE

A Foley catheter was inserted and there was no urine in the bladder. Over the next six hours, there was no urine output despite adequate hydration. A plain film of the abdomen revealed a staghorn calculus of the right kidney (Fig. 50.3). Infusion intravenous urogram revealed on early nephrogram. Subsequent films showed hydronephrosis to the level of the right ureteropelvic junction (Fig. 50.4). She was taken to the operating room, and a ureteral catheter was passed into the right renal pelvis with ease.

Renal Calculi   Case 50/ 241

Then she was placed in the lithotomy position and a right extended pyelolithotomy was performed without incident. Over the next several days, she had a brisk diuresis. In the following week, the blood urea nitrogen fell to 19mg% and the creatinine 1.1mg%. She was discharged on the 11th postoperative day. Follow-up films showed no evidence of residual calculi in the kidney (Fig. 50.5).

See Case 51 for Questions and References.

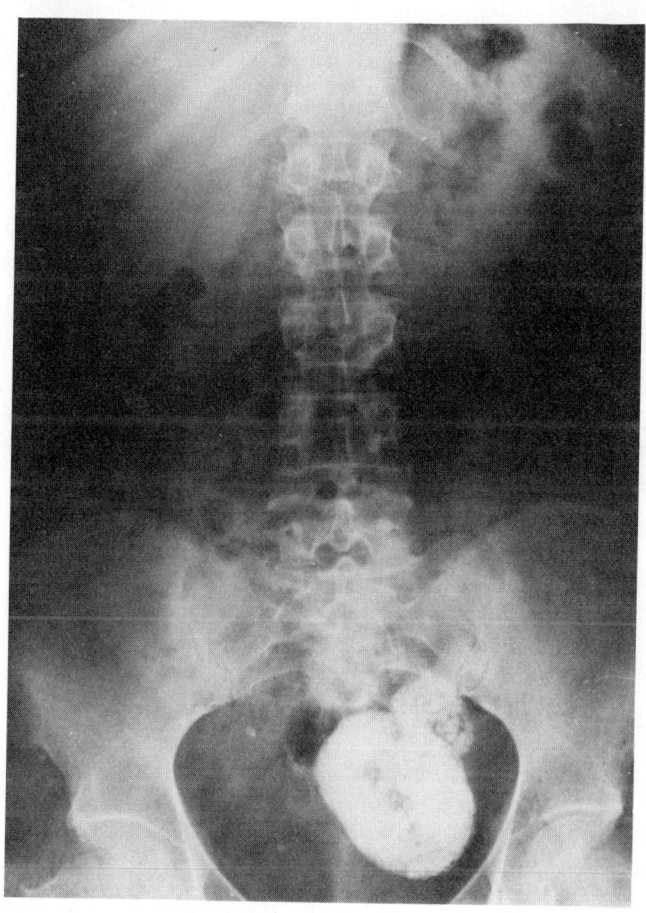

FIG. 50.1: Plain film of abdomen, November, 1977. No evidence of calculi.

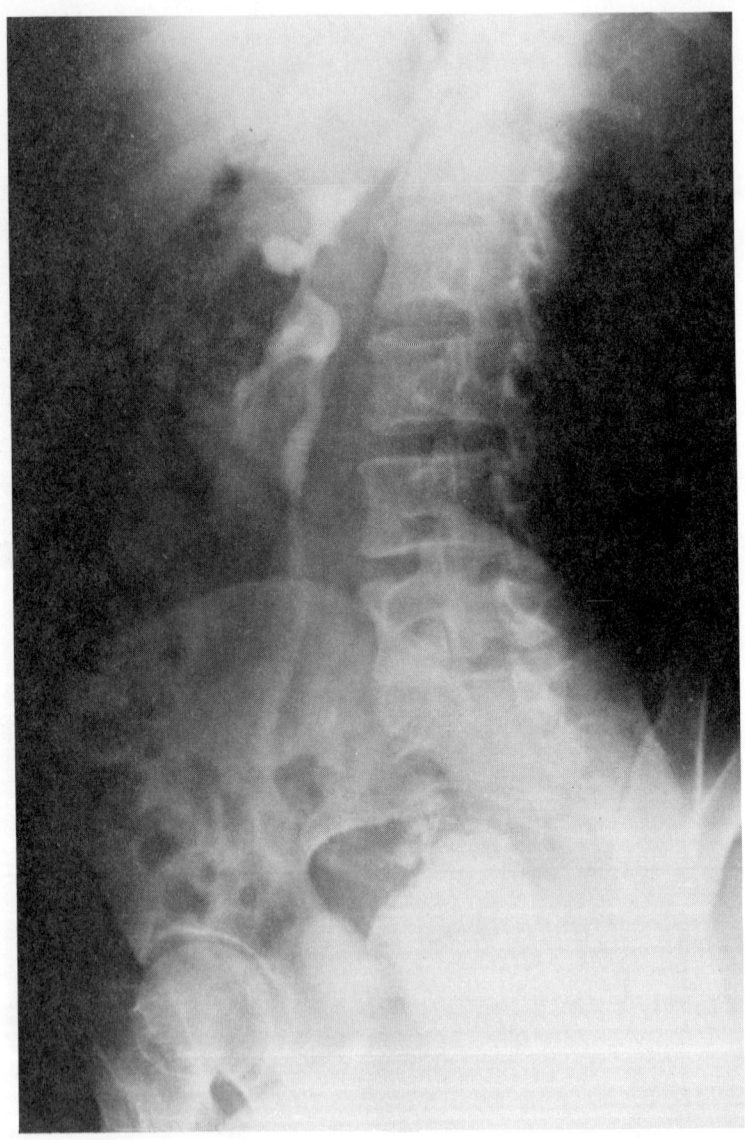

FIG. 50.2: Intravenous urogram, November, 1977 showing evidence of papillary necrosis in lower pole.

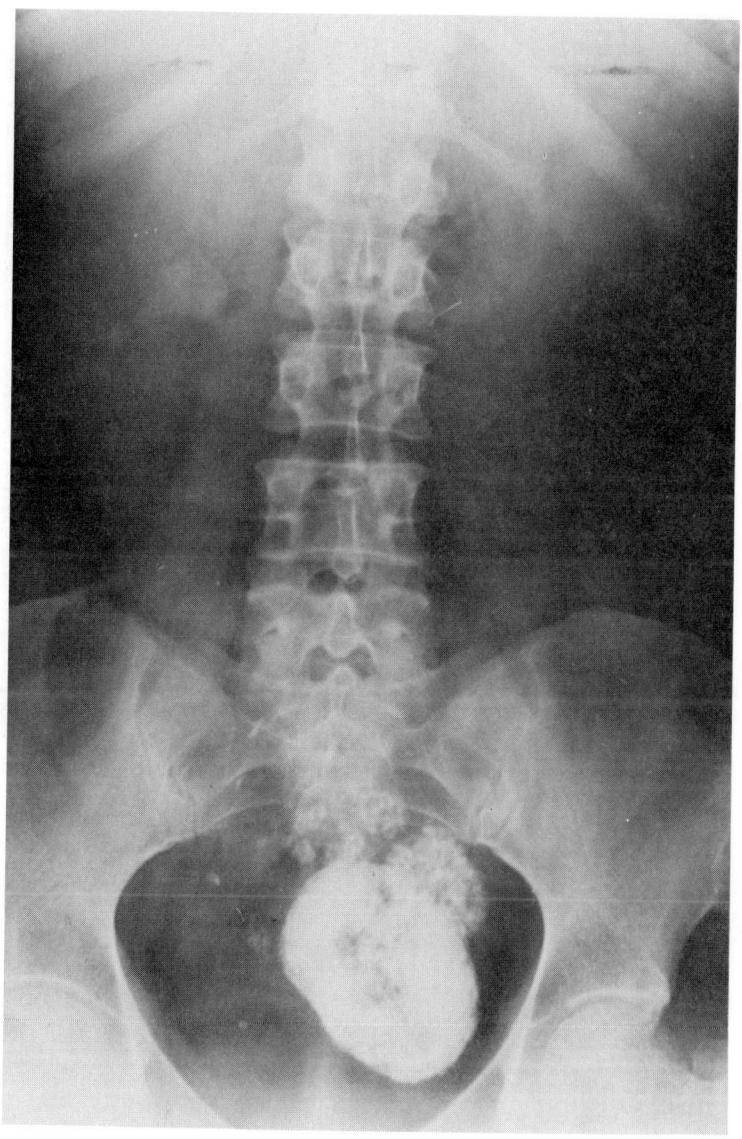

FIG. 50.3: Plain film of abdomen, February, 1978, showing staghorn calculus.

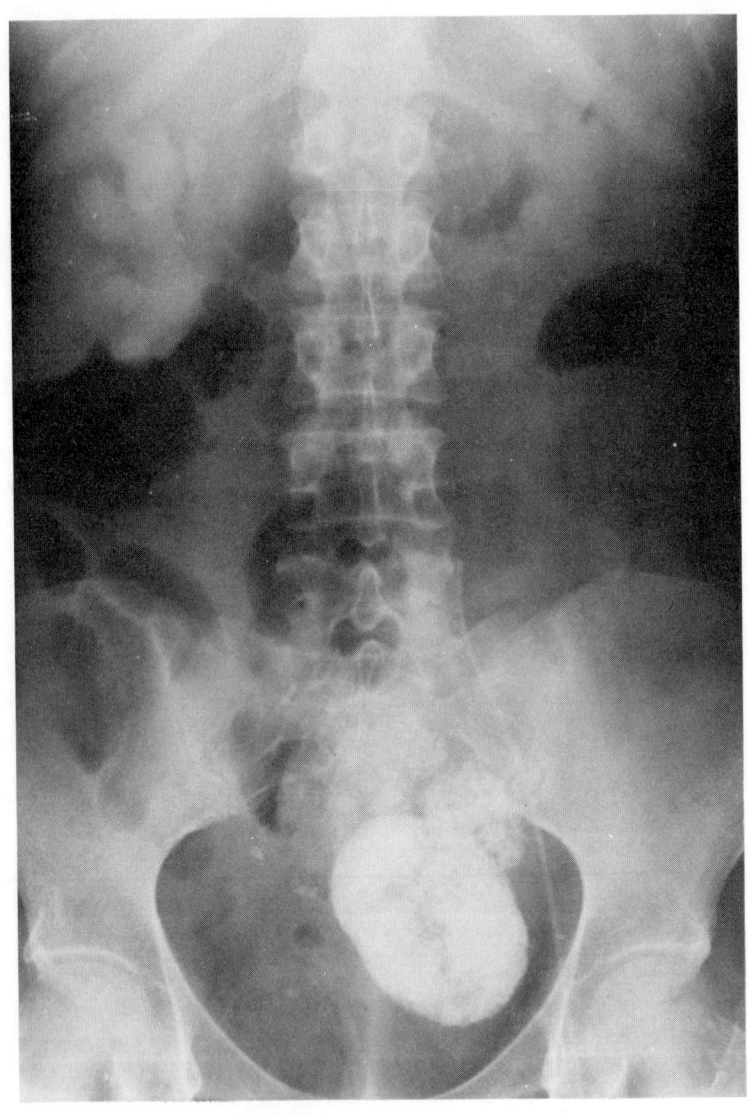

FIG. 50.4: Intravenous urogram.

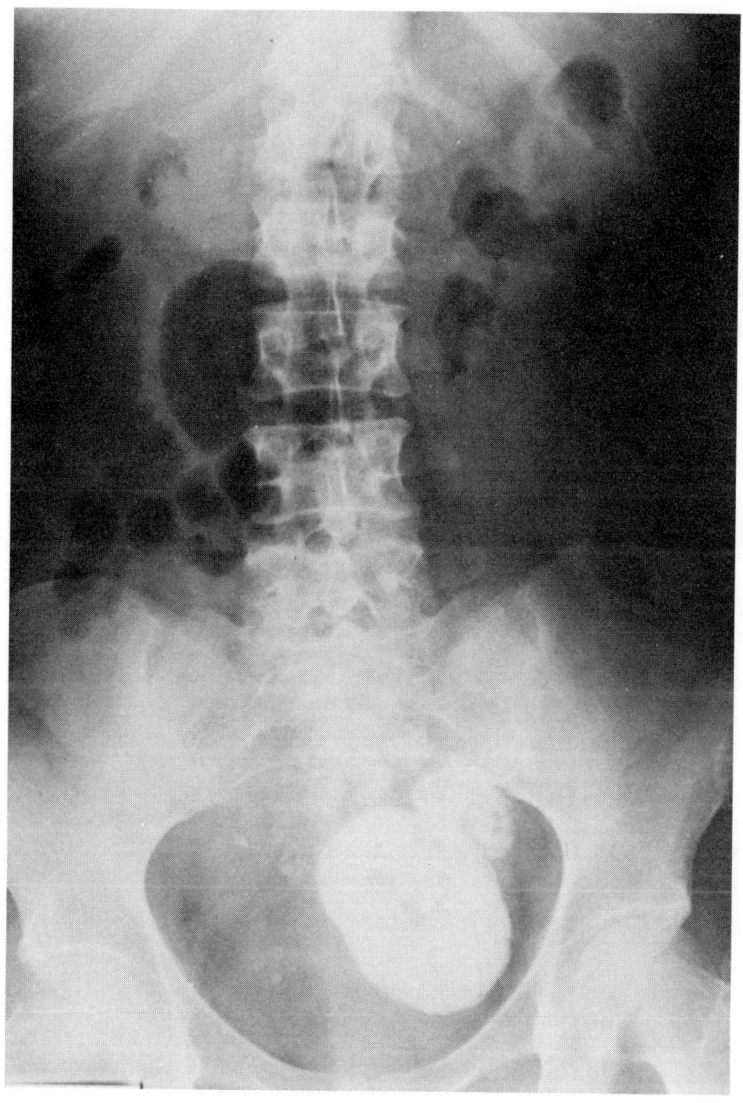

FIG. 50. 5: Plain film of abdomen six months after removal of calculus.

CASE 51: 26-YEAR-OLD FEMALE WITH HEMATURIA DURING PREGNANCY

HISTORY

A 26-year-old female was seen in her 31st week of pregnancy because of gross total painless hematuria. She denied frequency, urgency, dysuria, or back pain. There were no chills nor fever. The hematuria persisted on and off grossly for the next two weeks. It was elected to postpone urologic investigation until the postpartum period. She had an episode of acute right pyelonephritis in her 35th week of pregnancy, and she responded promptly to intravenous ampicillin and delivered a normal baby soon after this. She denied a family history of renal calculi.

PHYSICAL EXAMINATION

Blood pressure 110/70. There was no CVA tenderness. The abdomen was normal. After delivery, pelvic and rectal examination were normal.

LABORATORY DATA

Urine analysis: Many RBCs and many WBCs at the time of her episode of pyelonephritis. Urine culture at that time showed over 100,000 colonies of E. coli, but many subsequent cultures revealed no growth. A plain film of the abdomen revealed bilateral staghorn calculi (Fig. 51.1). There was prompt bilateral excretion on intravenous urography showing normal upper collecting systems and normal ureters (Fig. 51.2). Serum calcium, phosphorus and uric acid were all within normal limits on many determinations. Twenty-four hour urinary calcium, phosphorus and uric acid and cystine excretions were normal on numerous occasions. Kidney function studies were all within normal limits.

CLINICAL COURSE

Six weeks after delivery, she underwent removal of the right staghorn calculus through an extended pyelolithotomy. She had an uneventful postoperative course, and both intraoperative and postoperative films showed complete removal of the entire calculus. She did well after this and three months later underwent left nephro and pyelolithotomy. Following this, her postoperative course was entirely uneventful. A plain film of the abdomen after this procedure is shown in Fig. 51.3. An intravenous urogram six weeks after the second procedure is shown in Fig. 51.4. After her last procedure, she has done well for the past

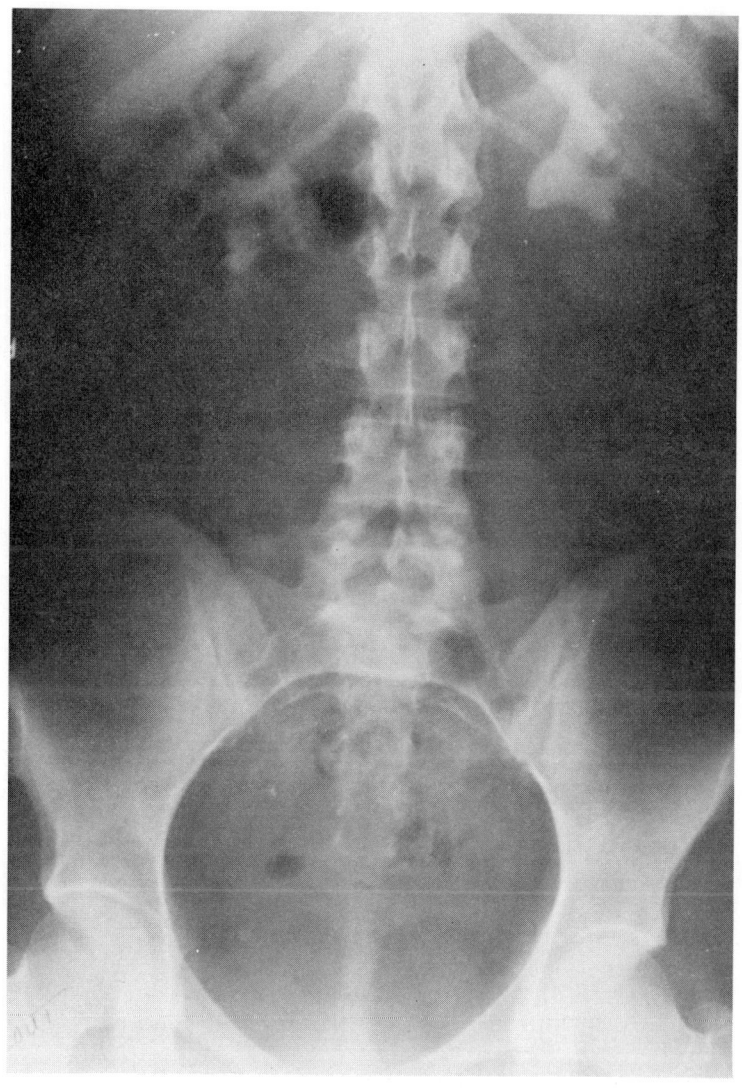

FIG. 51.1: Plain film of abdomen. There are bilateral staghorn calculi.

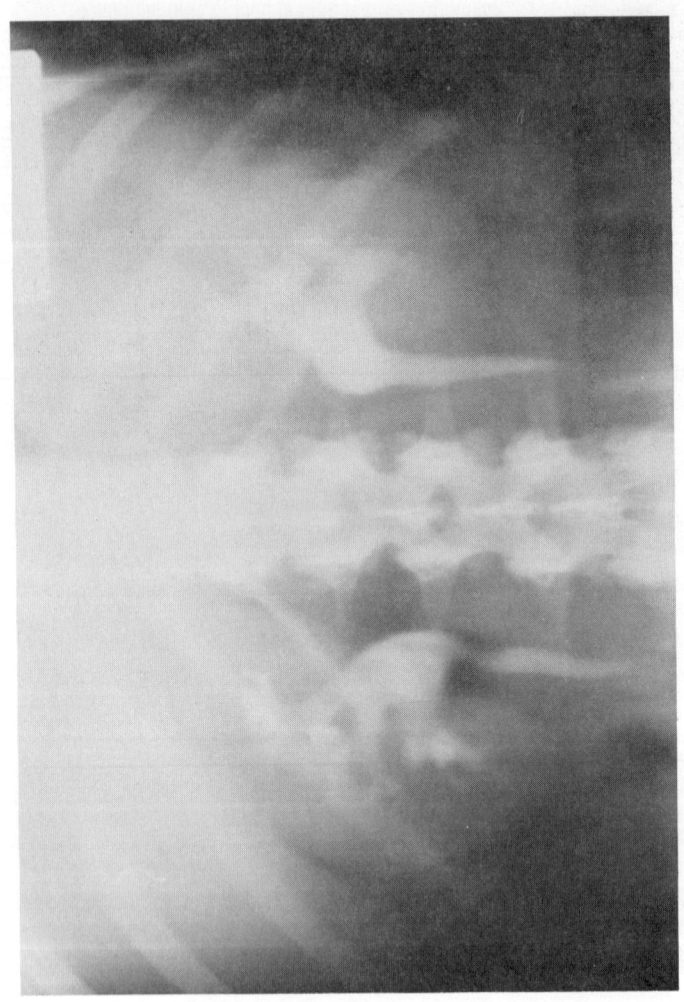

FIG. 51.2: Intravenous urogram showing normal upper tract.

Renal Calculi

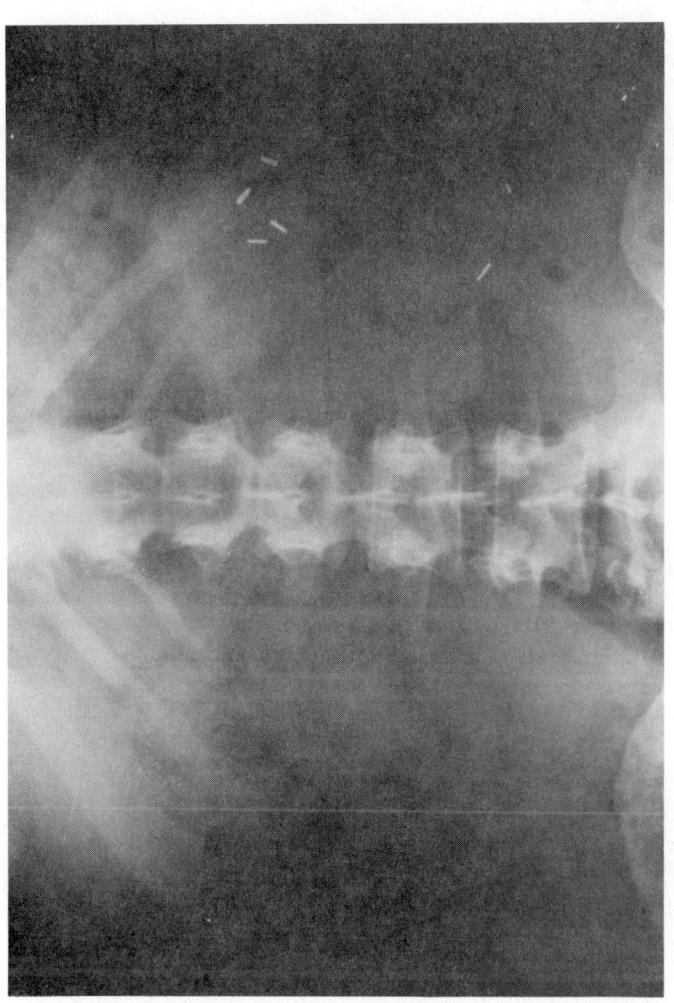

FIG. 51.3: Plain film of abdomen after removal of bilateral staghorn calculi.

250/ Case 51   Renal Calculi

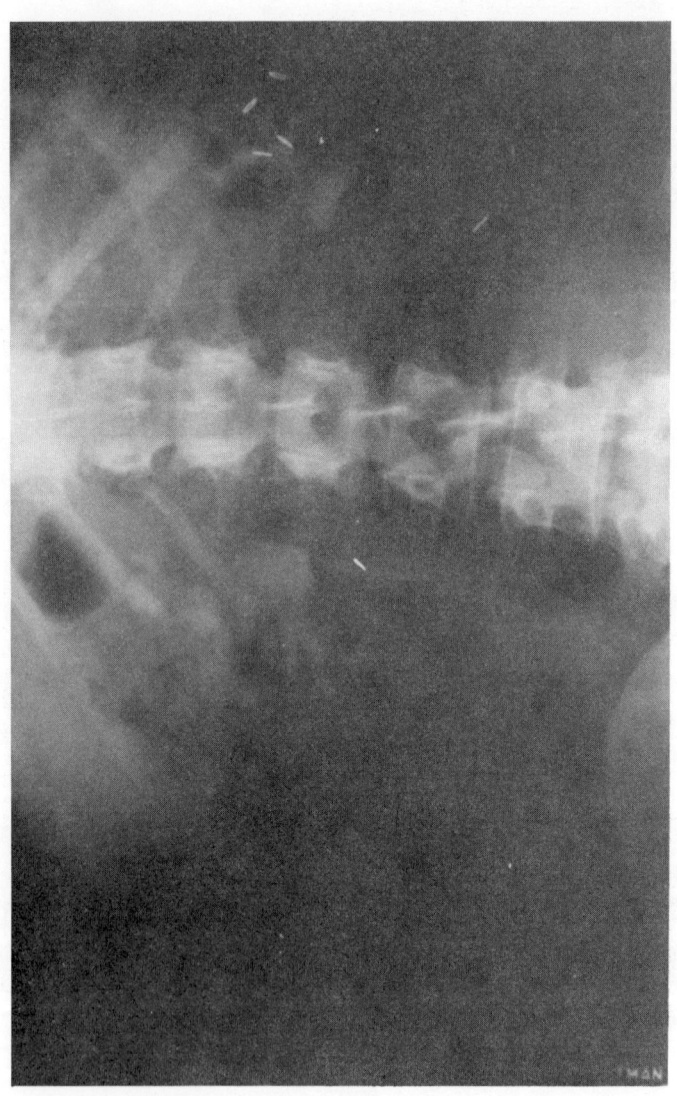

FIG. 51.4: Intravenous urogram 6 weeks after second procedure.

Renal Calculi

two years and has had a second and uneventful pregnancy. All urine cultures have remained sterile.

QUESTIONS: CASES 50-51

(T)RUE OR (F)ALSE:

1. Most staghorn calculi are asymptomatic.

2. Because most staghorn calculi are asymptomatic, it is better to leave them alone as long as there is no obstruction.

3. If not removed completely, a staghorn calculus always will recur.

4. If staghorn calculi are removed completely, they will recur most of the time.

5. In the presence of a staghorn calculus and a patient who is relatively well, it is better to remove the stone than to do a nephrectomy, and better to do a nephrectomy than to do nothing.

6. Most patients with staghorn calculi will have sterile urine.

7. The most common organism associated with staghorn calculi is E. coli.

8. Which of the following are not branches of the left main renal artery?
   A. Apical branch
   B. Adrenal
   C. Spermatic
   D. Posterior
   E. Anterior superior

9. The optimum temperature for cooling the kidney has been shown to be:
   A. $0°C$
   B. $5°C$
   C. $10°C$
   D. $20°C$
   E. $30°C$

10. If the renal artery is to be clamped without renal cooling, ischemia time should not exceed:
    A. 10 minutes
    B. 20 minutes

C. 30 minutes
D. 60 minutes
E. 120 minutes

11. The overall recurrence rate of calculi after removal of staghorn is:
    A. 5-10%
    B. 10-20%
    C. 20-30%
    D. 30-40%
    E. Over 50%

ANSWERS AND DISCUSSION: CASES 50-51

1. (F) The majority of patients with staghorn calculi are significantly symptomatic. In Blandy's series of more than 150 cases, 81.5% had pain, 48% had hematuria, and 79.4% had infection.

2. (F) As previously stated, most staghorn calculi are not asymptomatic and, if left alone, can cause significant symptoms and complicating problems. They also can lead to death by renal failure or by sepsis.

3. (F) If not removed completely, staghorn calculi will recur in about 30% of patients (in the larger series, as reported by Blandy and Boyce).

4. (F) If removed completely, the recurrence rate of staghorn calculi was 15% reported by Boyce, and 12.5% by Blandy.

5. (T) The preservation of renal function always should be uppermost in the urologist's mind and, if possible, pyelo or nephrolithotomy always is preferable to nephrectomy. Blandy has shown in his large series that patients who had "conservative" treatment, i.e., observation only, did much worse than those who had nephrectomy or removal of the calculus.

6. (F) In Boyce's series of 100 patients, only 33.3% had sterile urine.

7. (F) Proteus species comprised the majority of the positive cultures. E. coli, Pseudomonas and Klebsiella species were about equally represented in the remainder of the positive cultures found.

8. (C) Both spermatic arteries are branches of the aorta. The left spermatic vein drains into the left renal vein. The main

renal artery generally branches into an anterior and posterior branch. The apical branch can come off either one of these. The anterior branch then divides into an anterior superior, an anterior inferior, and the basilar branch.

9. (D) Wickham has shown that the optimum temperature for renal cooling is $20^{\circ}C$. The renal artery can be kept clamped easily for two or three hours at this temperature with complete return of renal function.

10. (C) In the same experimental work as previously mentioned, it was shown that once warm ischemia time exceeded 30 minutes, there was significant and irreversible renal damage.

11. (B) As previously stated, the overall recurrence rate of staghorn calculi in Boyce's series was 15% and in Blandy's series, it was reported as 12.5%.

REFERENCES: CASES 50-51

1. Singh MR, et al.: The fate of the unoperated staghorn calculus. Brit J Urol 45:581-585, 1973.

2. Singh M, Tresidder GC, and Blandy J: The long-term results of removal of staghorn calculi by extended pyelolithotomy without cooling or renal artery occlusion. Brit J Urol 43:658-664, 1971.

3. Boyce WH and Elkins IB: Reconstructive renal surgery following anatrophic nephrolithotomy: Follow-up of 100 consecutive cases. J Urol 111:307, 1974.

4. Wickham JEA, Hanley HG, and Joekes AM: Regional renal hypothermia. Brit J Urol 39:727, 1967.

5. Boyce WH: Chapter 12. In: Urologic Surgery, Glenn SF (ed.), Harper & Row, New York, 1975.

CASE 52: 65-YEAR-OLD MALE WITH DYSURIA AND FREQUENCY

HISTORY

A 65-year-old male was seen because of dysuria and frequency of urination every half hour, day and night. He stated he had been passing small stones per urethra for months.

PHYSICAL EXAMINATION

The blood pressure was 170/100. Heart and chest were normal. Abdomen was normal. On rectal examination, the prostate was 2 to 3x enlarged, smooth, firm, and nontender with well-defined boundaries.

LABORATORY DATA

A urinalysis showed gross pyuria and many red cells. CBC, BUN and FBS were normal. ECG and chest x-ray normal. Plain film of the abdomen showed a kyphoscoliosis of the lumbar spine with discrete and confluent radiopacities occupying a circular area in the bony pelvis approximately 6cm in diameter (Fig. 52.1).

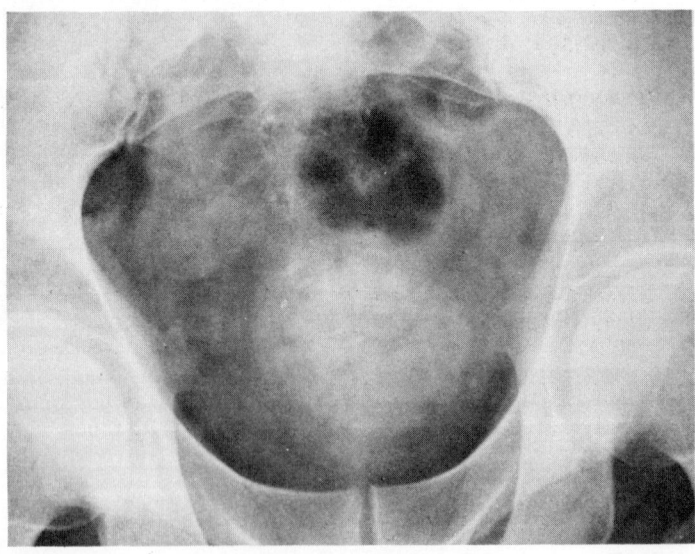

FIG. 52.1: Plain film of the abdomen showing numerous bladder calculi.

Renal Calculi

The excretory urogram demonstrated partial opacification of the dilated calyces bilaterally in good concentration, and a one-hour film revealed ureterectasia down to the ureterovesical junction with tortuosity (Fig. 52.2). The bladder was opacified around the stones and numerous diverticulae were noted. Urine culture showed E. coli sensitive to most antibiotics.

QUESTIONS

1. The composition of the stones in this case is most likely:
    A. Calcium oxalate
    B. Cystine
    C. Magnesium ammonium phosphate
    D. Uric acid
    E. Calcium phosphate

2. The optimum management of this patient would be:
    A. Treatment with most potent antibiotic; when urine is sterile, remove the stones and prostate.
    B. Remove the stones and prostate in one stage and then treat with antibiotics.
    C. Remove the stones in one stage, perform prostatectomy as a second stage, and then treat the infection.
    D. Remove only the stones, treat the infection and then re-evaluate regarding prostatectomy.

3. Bladder calculi in the United States are usually:
    A. Secondary to infection
    B. Secondary to obstruction
    C. Secondary to enlarged stones originally passed from the kidney
    D. Primary stones formed in the bladder secondary to metabolic defects

CLINICAL COURSE

A suprapubic cystolithotomy and evacuation of the diverticuli of stone was performed as a first stage operation, leaving the patient with a suprapubic cystostomy tube in place. Twelve days later, a second stage suprapubic prostatectomy was performed and the patient made an uneventful recovery. The stones were magnesium ammonium phosphate.

ANSWERS AND DISCUSSION

1. (C) The stones are radiopaque, and therefore, uric acid calculus is omitted immediately. Stones in the bladder, in the

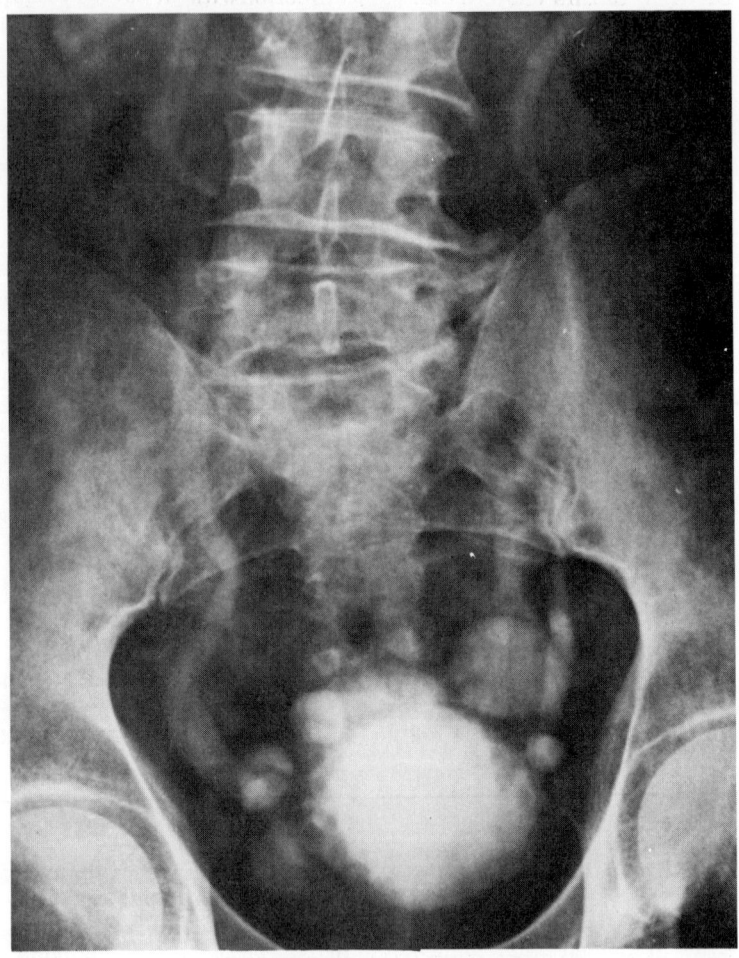

FIG. 52.2: A one-hour film revealing ureterectasia down to the ureterovesical junction with tortuosity.

Renal Calculi   Case 52/ 257

presence of infection, usually are magnesium ammonium phosphate. Although proteus species generally are associated with these, any gram negative organism may be involved.

2. (C) In this case, treating the infection without surgery would be folly because of the presence of infected stones, as well as urinary obstruction. The safest method of management would be removal of the stones and cystostomy, followed by second stage prostatectomy. Performing all these procedures simultaneously runs the risk of sepsis, with opening of the venous channels at the time of prostatectomy. Although, with the potent antibiotics available today, this easily could be done as a one-stage procedure, there certainly is added risk in doing this.

3. (B) Most bladder calculi in the United States are secondary to obstruction. Infection may accompany the process, but the majority of stones are not associated with infection. Invariably, the obstruction has to be treated as well as the calculus.

CASE 53: 56-YEAR-OLD FEMALE WITH FREQUENCY AND DYSURIA

HISTORY

A 56-year-old female was seen because of frequency of urination, as well as dysuria. In the past, she had had numerous urinary tract infections. She also complained of dyspareunia.

PHYSICAL EXAMINATION

A markedly obese female. There were no abdominal masses. External genitalia were normal. Vaginal examination revealed a rock-hard, smooth mass in the anterior wall of the vagina; it was quite tender. Speculum exam revealed an ulceration of the anterior vaginal wall through which a large stone could be seen (Fig. 53.1).

LABORATORY DATA

Urinalysis revealed many WBC and many RBC per high power field. Culture showed more than 100,000 colonies E. coli sensitive to most antibiotics tested. Blood count revealed WBC 12,000 with a left shift. Blood urea nitrogen and creatinine were normal. ECG and chest x-ray were normal. Abdominal film showed a calcification in the pelvis measuring 3.5cm in diameter (Fig. 53.2). After injection of contrast material, the upper tracts were normal. Retrograde cystogram revealed a large urethral diverticulum; the stone was in this diverticulum (Fig. 53.3).

HOSPITAL COURSE

After the previously mentioned studies were carried out, the patient was taken to the operating room and the large calculus removed vaginally. The urethral diverticulum was excised to its base, and the defect in the urethra was closed in two layers with interrupted 3.0 chromic catgut sutures. A Foley catheter was left in place for 10 days, after which the patient voided with good control. She has had several recurrent bouts of acute cystitis since surgery, but between these bouts, her urine remains sterile. A repeat cystourethrogram is normal.

QUESTIONS

1. All of the following are etiologic factors in formation of urethral diverticulum, except:

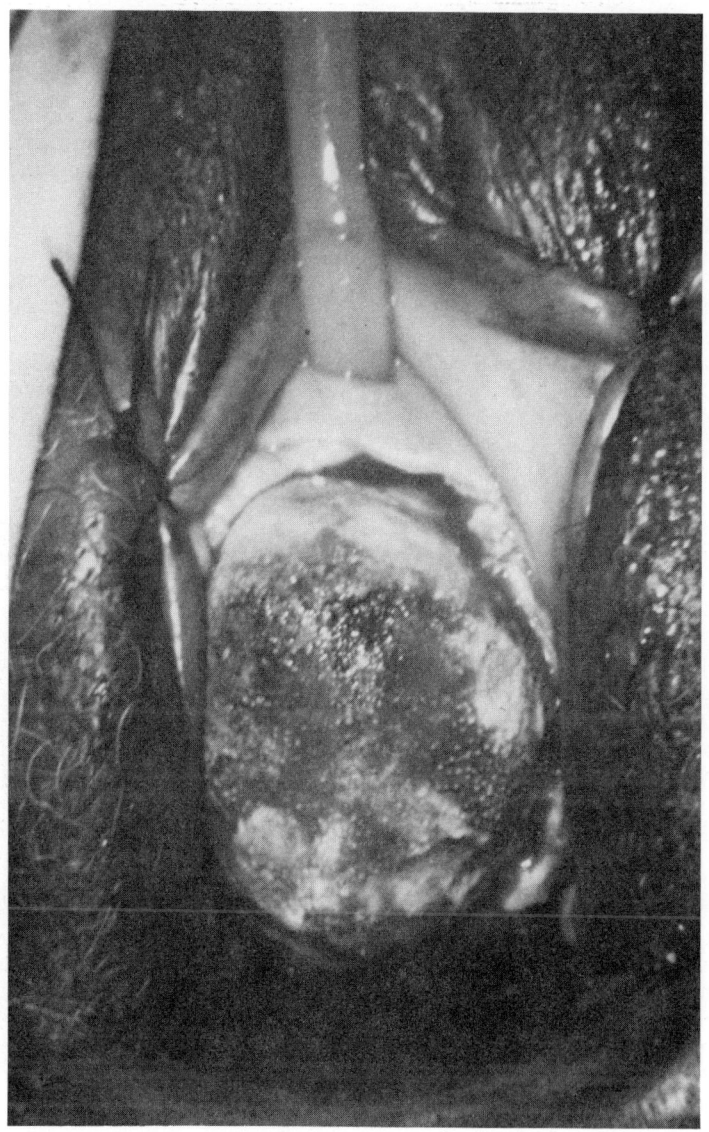

FIG. 53.1: Ulceration of anterior vaginal wall through which a large stone can be seen.

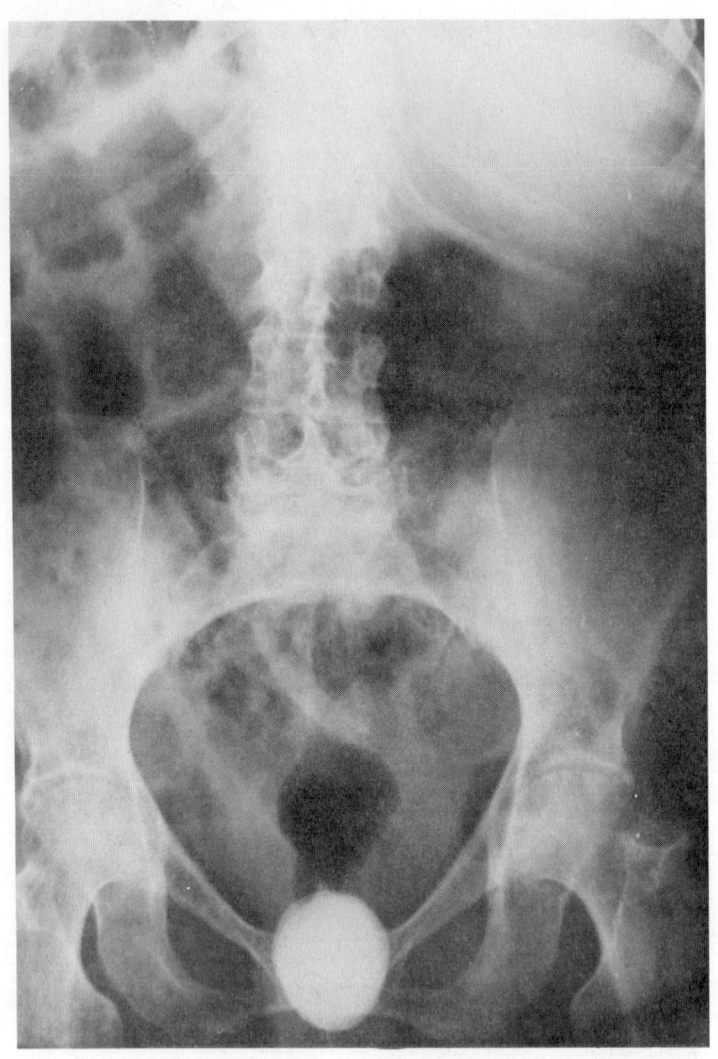

FIG. 53.2: KUB showing large calculus.

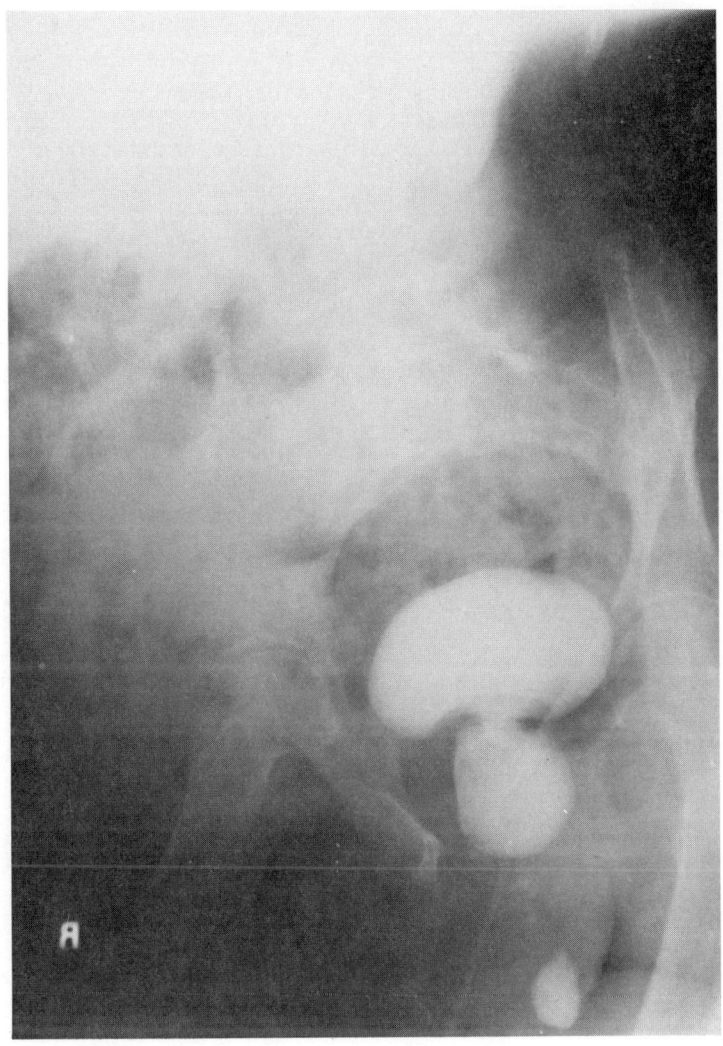

FIG. 53.3: Retrograde cystogram showing urethral diverticulum.

A. Obstetric urethral trauma
B. Recurrent urethral infection
C. Periurethral abscess
D. Congenital
E. Passage of a calculus

2. Which of the following is the most significant symptom of urethral diverticulum?
   A. Urethral discharge on compression of the urethra
   B. Dyspareunia
   C. Recurrent cystitis
   D. Tenderness over the urethra
   E. All of the above

(T)RUE OR (F)ALSE

3. The opening of urethral diverticulum usually be seen cystoscopically.

ANSWERS AND DISCUSSION

1. (E) Most diverticulae of the urethra are secondary to chronic infection of the periurethral glands, with cyst and abscess formation, and finally rupture into the urethra. Obstetrical trauma to the periurethral area may account for some diverticulae, but this is probably rare. Congenital diverticulae of the urethra do occur and usually present in childhood. For calculus lodging in the urethra to later develop into a diverticulum would be most unlikely.

2. (E) Dyspareunia associated with recurrent urinary tract infection and urinary symptoms always should alert one to the possibility of a urethral diverticulum. Expressable pus from the urethra is a significant finding, as is tenderness over the urethra, but it is commonly seen in urethritis secondary to any source. A palpable cystic mass in the area of the urethra would also be highly indicative of a urethral diverticulum.

3. (F) The urethral opening of the diverticulum may be very small and not easily visualized. Borski and Stutsman have described a method of visualization. The diverticulum is emptied by manual compression per vagina. A catheter is passed into the bladder and the bladder filled with saline solution containing indigo carmine. The patient is asked to void while in the lithotomy position. As she voids the examiner partially occludes the urethral meatus with the finger.

This allows the diverticulum to fill with the dye-colored fluid. Urethroscopy then is performed, and the blue stained fluid can then be seen coming from the diverticular opening. The diverticulum may be demonstrated radiologically by the use of the Davis-Te Linde double lumened catheter.

CHAPTER X

THE ADRENAL GLAND

INTRODUCTION

The adrenal gland has been of great interest to the urologist because of its location in the retroperitoneum, adjacent to the kidney, and because localization of surgical disease of the adrenal traditionally has been accomplished by urologic methods.

The gland is of dual origin embryologically; the cortex being derived from gonadotropic mesoderm and the medulla from sympathetic neuroectoderm. The cortex is divided into three zones - the glomerular zone, fascicular zone and reticular zone. Each zone is believed to give rise to different classes of adrenal hormones - the outer, glomerular zone forming the mineralocorticoids, the fascicular zone giving rise to the glucocorticoids, and the reticular zone forming the various 17 ketosteroids. Hyperfunction of the adrenal cortex may be due to hyperplasia or neoplasia. In the former, both glands are hyperactive and enlarged. In the latter, hyperfunction is secondary to a tumor - which may be malignant or benign. Neoplasms of the adrenal generally can be localized by the methods illustrated in Case 54. Hyperfunction of the adrenal may give rise to adrenogenital syndrome, Cushing's syndrome, or hyperaldosteronism.

The adrenal medulla consists of two types of cells: 1) the sympathocytes which receive stimuli from the sympathetic innervation and control pheochromocyte activity; and 2) pheochromocytes which elaborate epinephrine and norepinephrine. Sympathocytes give rise to three types of tumors: 1) sympathicoblastoma; 2) intermediate cell type neuroblastoma, and 3) ganglioneuroma. The pheochromocytes give rise to the neoplasm of pheochromocytoma illustrated in Cases 55 and 56.

CASE 54: 40-YEAR-OLD FEMALE WITH HYPERTENSION AND AMENORRHEA

HISTORY

A 40-year-old white married female presented typical symptoms of Cushing's syndrome - centripetal obesity; moon facies; facial hirsutism; easy bruisability; thinness of skin; amenorrhea; supraclavicular fat pads; recent onset of hypertension; muscular weakness; and some back pain. All symptoms had appeared over the last $1\frac{1}{2}$-2 years.

PHYSICAL EXAMINATION

Blood pressure was 200/100. The patient had typical appearance of Cushing's syndrome with a somewhat plethoric face, a few telangiectatic veins and definite "chipmunk" configuration to the facies. There were very prominent supraclavicular fat pads, without a prominent cervicodorsal hymp. The skin was paper thin and bruise marks were seen scattered over the extremities. There was a violatious hue to the legs which appeared inordinately thin in relation to the trunk.

LABORATORY DATA: Routine studies were all normal.

	Base Line	p Dexameth 0.75 t.i.d.	p Dexameth 2.25 t.i.d.
17 ketosteroids	12 mg/24 hr	10mg	10
17 ketogenic steroids	22mg/24 hr	21mg	22
		Before ACTH	After ACTH
170 Hcorticosteroids		19 micrograms	39 micrograms

The fact that all routine studies were normal indicates a normal response.

The interpretation of the above was that the patient had a non-suppressable adrenal tumor. In order to localize the tumor, an arteriogram was performed, which was normal. Presacral CO_2 insufflation revealed an enlarged left adrenal and no apparent tissue on the right. Nephrotomography, with a mass above the left kidney, is shown in Fig. 54.1.

266/ Case 54   The Adrenal Gland

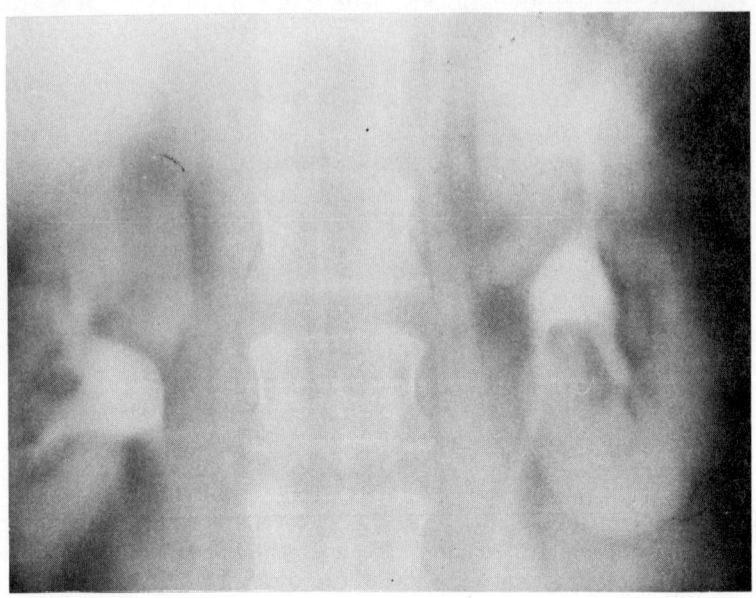

FIG. 54.1: Nephrotomography showing a mass above the left kidney.

The patient was operated on through a left flank incision, removing the 12th rib. A left adrenal tumor weighing 12 grams was removed; it was well-encapsulated and histologically benign.

Prior to surgery, the patient was treated with 300mg a day of cortisone acetate. During surgery an intravenous drip of hydrocortisone was given. Steroids were tapered gradually, and she failed to develop symptoms. She had a spontaneous menses immediately post-op and all previously mentioned signs of Cushing's had disappeared by the third postoperative month.

QUESTIONS

1. The adrenal gland receives its blood supply from:
    A. The aorta
    B. The renal artery
    C. The inferior phrenic artery
    D. All of the above
    E. None of the above

The Adrenal Gland

2. The adrenal cortex arises from:
   A. Mesoderm
   B. Entoderm
   C. Endoderm

3. All of the following are precursors of cortisol production, except:
   A. Cholesterol
   B. Pregnenolone
   C. Progesterone
   D. Corticosterone
   E. 11-deoxycortisol

(T)RUE OR (F)ALSE:

4. Cushing's syndrome occurs more often in females.

5. When found in children or patients over 50 years of age, the incidence of malignancy increases.

6. Secondary Cushing's syndrome due to intake of exogenous steroids is probably more common than primary Cushing's disease due to excess cortisol production.

7. Failure to suppress steroid production after low and high dose dexamethasone is indicative of adrenal tumor.

8. The best method of radiographic demonstration of an adrenal tumor today is:
   A. Renal artery angiography
   B. Nephrotomography
   C. Adrenal venography
   D. Presacral CO_2 insufflation

ANSWERS AND DISCUSSION

1. (D) The arterial supply of the adrenal gland is derived from the inferior phrenic arteries, the abdominal aorta, and the renal arteries. These three then divide into numerous small branches to supply the gland and must be dissected carefully at surgery.

2. (A) The adrenal cortex arises embryologically from mesodermal cells at the cranial end of the mesonephros. The cells differentiate into the three zones described in the introduction to this section.

3. (D) Corticosterone is a precursor of the "mineralocorticoid" aldosterone. ACTH stimulates the adrenal to form pregnelone from cholesterol, which is then dehydrogenated to progesterone. The latter then can be converted to testosterone or 11-deoxycortisol by 21 hydroxylase. 11-deoxycortisol then is converted into cortisol, the active "glucocorticoid."

4. (T) Over 70% of Cushing's syndrome result from ACTH
5. (T) dependence.
6. (T)
7. (T)

8. (C) The multiple arterial supply of the adrenal makes adrenal arteriography difficult. Retroperitoneal CO_2 insufflation often is difficult to interpret and can be hazardous. The best method of study is adrenal venography - these veins are relatively easy to cannulate. This also allows collection of adrenal venous blood for analysis of steroid excretion. CTT scan would be most helpful.

CASE 55: 41-YEAR-OLD FEMALE WITH HYPERTENSION

HISTORY

A 41-year-old female was seen in the hypertension clinic because of a recent onset of blood pressure of 160-180/94-110. She complained of intermittent episodes of headache and palpitation associated with sweating, nausea, and vomiting. She stated she was always a "fidgety and nervous type individual." There was a 10-pound weight loss over the last year.

PHYSICAL EXAMINATION

A thin, very nervous individual. Blood pressure was 160/100. Heart, chest, abdomen, pulses were all within normal limits. Pelvic examination was normal.

LABORATORY DATA

A normal CBC, urinalysis and culture. VDRL was negative. Sedimentation rate 20 mm/hr. An intravenous urogram was entirely within normal limits. After 5mg of phentolamine intravenously, the blood pressure fell to 130/86 from a baseline of 154-160/100-104 and then gradually rose to baseline levels. Twenty-four-hour urinary vanillylmandelic acid (VMA) was 22mg.

CLINICAL COURSE

The patient underwent transperitoneal exploration. The adrenals were exposed first and appeared normal. A small tumor (1.5 x 2.0 cms) was palpated just superior to the right renal artery and removed. Following this, the blood pressure immediately fell to 80/60, but responded rapidly to plasma expanders and blood. Her postoperative course was uneventful and her blood pressure has been normal for one year postoperatively.

QUESTIONS

1. The classic symptoms triad of pheochromocytoma is:
    A. Hypertension, nervousness, and diabetes
    B. Sweating, palpitation, and headache
    C. Hypertension, headache, and nervousness
    D. Nervousness, ruddy complexion, and diarrhea

2. The optimum exposure for pheochromocytoma would be:
    A. Thoracoabdominal
    B. Classical flank

C. Through the 12th rib
D. Anterior transperitoneal midline

3. The following sometimes are associated with pheochromocytoma:
   A. von Recklinghausen's disease
   B. von Hippel-Lindau's disease
   C. Medullary thyroid carcinoma
   D. All of the above
   E. None of the above

4. The following drugs may be indicated in the preoperative preparation of a patient with pheochromocytoma:
   A. Alpha-adrenergic blocking agents
   B. Beta-adrenergic blocking agents
   C. Plasma volume expanders
   D. All of the above
   E. None of the above

5. Localization of a pheochromocytoma can be accomplished best by:
   A. Intravenous urography
   B. Renal angiography
   C. Vena caval catheterization
   D. Adrenal venography
   E. Sonography

ANSWERS AND DISCUSSION

1. (B) With careful history, one usually can elicit the classic triad of sweating, palpitations, and headaches in most patients. Although hypertension usually is the presenting symptom, the above generally are found as well.

2. (D) Pheochromocytomas occasionally are multiple or extra-adrenal, and, therefore, the flank approach or similar incisions would limit severely the complete exploration of the abdomen. The optimum approach would be one that affords complete abdominal exploration.

3. (D) All of those mentioned may be associated with pheochromocytoma. Both von Recklinghausen's and von Hippel-Lindau's disease have been reported in association with pheochromocytoma. The multiple endocrine adenoma syndrome is characterized by hyperparathyroidism, thyroid medullary carcinoma and pheochromocytoma. The latter may be

The Adrenal Gland   Case 55/ 271

multiple in this syndrome. This appears to be different from the pituitary-pancreas and parathyroid multiple adenoma syndrome.

4. (D) All of the agents may be useful. The alpha adrenergic blocking agents - Regitine and Dibenzyline may be used to lower excessive blood pressure levels in the preoperative period. Propanalol, a beta-adrenergic blocking agent, may be necessary for cardiac arrhythmias often associated with this disease. Decreased plasma volume secondary to the marked peripheral vasoconstriction also accompanies the disease. This may be corrected by alpha-adrenergic agent, but frequently plasma expanders must be used as well.

5. (E) Vena caval catheterization, with blood sampling at various levels, is a method for localizing extra-adrenal tumors preoperatively. Sonography is probably the best method generally available today. With more extensive use of CAT Scans, this may add further to an accurate preoperative localization of the tumor.

CASE 56: 79-YEAR-OLD FEMALE WITH NAUSEA, VOMITING AND ABDOMINAL MASS

HISTORY

A 79-year-old female was admitted because of episodes of nausea, vomiting, and abdominal fullness. She had been tested for "peptic ulcer" and "diverticulosis" with temporary relief. She had had an appendectomy, herniorrhaphy, cholecystectomy, and hysterectomy in the past. She denied a history of hypertension, cardiac disease, diabetes, and neoplasia in herself or her family. She denied attacks of sweating.

PHYSICAL EXAMINATION

Blood Pressure: Supine 160/10; Upright 110/60. There was moderate obesity. No cardiopulmonary abnormality. There was an ill-defined mass in the right upper quadrant separate from the liver and not moving with respiration.

LABORATORY DATA

Hct: 45%. Blood Sugar: 130-140mg%. An intravenous urogram revealed a large mass in the upper pole of the right kidney - possibly adrenal in origin (Fig. 56.1). Aortography and selective renal angiography showed the mass to be adrenal in origin and probably representing a pheochromocytoma (Fig, 56.2). Total Serum Catecholamine: 2933 P.G./ml (normal = 120-465). 24-hour urine:

a) Total catecholamine 425mcg.
    epinephrine 349mcg.
b) Vanillylmandelic acid 6.8mgm.
c) Metanephrine 4.1mgm

HOSPITAL COURSE

A midline incision was performed and the adrenal mass was removed uneventfully. Pathological diagnosis: malignant pheochromocytoma. The patient made an uneventful recovery. To date, seven months postoperatively, she is doing well without evidence of metastasis or recurrence.

QUESTIONS

1. The blood supply to the adrenal gland is derived from:
   A. The aorta

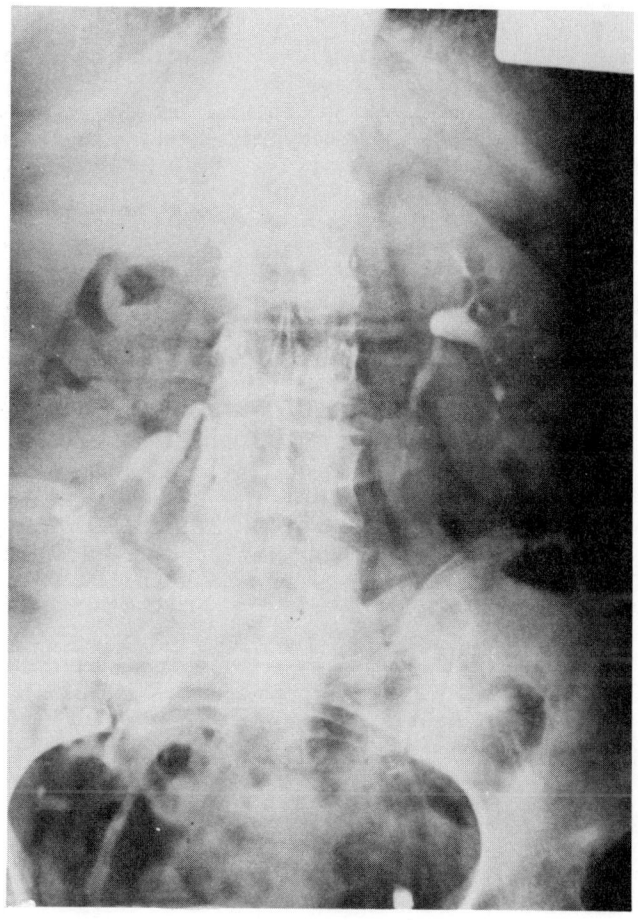

FIG. 56.1: Intravenous urogram revealing large mass in the upper pole of the right kidney.

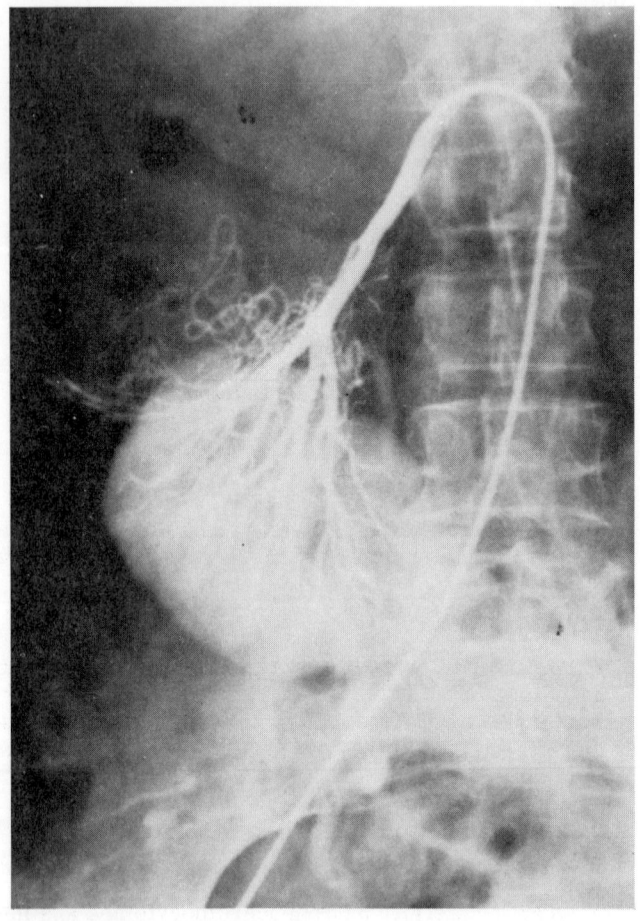

FIG. 56.2: Selective renal angiography showing mass to be adrenal in origin and probably representing a pheochromocytoma.

The Adrenal Gland   Case 56/ 275

    B. The inferior phrenic artery
    C. The renal artery
    D. All of the above
    E. None of the above

2. Which of the following is not a common area for development of "ecoptic" (extra-adrenal) pheochromocytoma:
    A. Anterior to right renal artery
    B. Anterior to bifurcation of the aorta
    C. The bladder
    D. The testicle

(T)RUE OR (F)ALSE:

3. The alpha blockers, phentomaline and phenoxybenzamine, are given preoperatively because the alpha effects of the catecholamines are predominant.

4. The patient with pheochromocytoma generally has excessive vascular volume and a high hematocrit.

5. The best method of preoperative localization of the tumor is by angiography.

6. If a pheochromocytoma definitely can be located in one adrenal, the preferred approach would be through a flank incision.

ANSWERS AND DISCUSSION

1. (D) The arterial supply to the adrenal could be variable, but usually is supplied from three sources. The superior adrenal artery is a branch of the inferior phrenic; the middle comes directly from the aorta and the inferior adrenal artery is derived from the renal artery on that side. The venous drainage is less variable, the main adrenal vein on the right emptying into the vena cava and on the left into the left renal vein.

2. (D) Approximately 15% of pheochromocytomas are multiple and 10% are extra-adrenal. The most common site is at the bifurcation of the aorta in the "organ of Zuckerkandel." The urinary bladder as a site of pheochromocytoma was first reported by Zimmerman in 1953. Since that time, numerous reports have appeared in the literature about other cases in this organ. The upper paraortic area is also involved commonly by extra-adrenal pheochromocytoma.

3. (T) The alpha effects of the catecholamines produced by
4. (F) the adrenal are the predominant ones and are responsible for both the severe hypertension and reduced vascular volume. Both of these are secondary to severe peripheral vasoconstriction. The reason for using alpha blockers preoperatively is because of their competitive inhibition of norepinephrine effects at the peripheral receptors.

5. (F) Once the diagnosis of pheochromocytoma has been established by clinical history and laboratory findings of elevated catecholamines or their by-products, the best method of localization of the tumor is by sonography or CAT Scan. Rather than relying on surgical exploration, this method accomplishes precise localization. Bone subtraction films may add to the precise localization of the tumor.

6. (F) Since as many as 15% of pheochromocytomas can be multiple and the great majority of them occur below the diaphragm, the accepted method of approach would be through an anterior transperitoneal incision. The flank incision would not allow further exploration of the abdominal cavity.

REFERENCES

1. Urol Clinics N Amer, Vol. 4, No. 2, W.B. Saunders Company, June 1977.

2. Gitlow SE, et al.: Pheochromocytoma - surgical aspects. Annals of Surgery 169:376-385, 1969.

3. Fernandez M: Management of patient with pheochromocytoma. Hospital Practice 4:43-47, 1976.

4. Zimmerman IJ, et al.: Pheochromocytoma of the urinary bladder. New Eng. J. Med. 249:25, 1953.

CHAPTER XI

NEUROGENIC BLADDER

INTRODUCTION

Vesical contraction is dependent upon an intact neural pathway involving sacral segments 2, 3, and 4 via the sacral nerve. The main motor nerve of the bladder is the parasympathetic nerve emanating from these segments. The bladder is also rich in sympathetic fibers. Sensory fibers leave the bladder, and travel with sympathetic, parasympathetic and somatic nerves entering the spinal cord at levels from T9 to S4 and ascending in the lateral spinothalamic tract and fasciculus gracilis. Vesical function is controlled by a spinal reflex mediated through the parasympathetic sacral segments mentioned above. Voluntary control of this reflex is mediated via the cerebral cortex.

Spinal cord bladder dysfunction can be divided into two main types: a) sacral lesions - those involving nerves at or below the parasympathetic outflow center of the bladder at S2, 3, and 4, and b) suprasacral lesions - those above the level of this center.

Lesions of the spinal cord above the sacral segments can be caused by various etiologic factors, most commonly trauma; but infection, primary or secondary tumors, or primary spinal cord disease, are other examples. Initially, in this type of neurogenic bladder, there is a period of hypotonicity with overflow incontinence and reflex voiding. The ability to initiate and terminate micturition is lost. Later, "trigger areas" may develop. Stroking of the leg or pressure on the penis initiate micturition. Voiding usually is interrupted and incomplete. Later, the detrusor becomes markedly hypertrophic and vesicoureteral reflux often develops. One sees the typical "Christmas tree" deformity. Suprasacral lesions are characterized by decreased capacity, involuntary contractions, high intravesical pressure and marked hypertrophy.

Lesions of the cauda equina and conus medullaris may be secondary to trauma, spina bifida and neoplasm. Here, there is an interruption of the reflex, and a loss of feeling of fullness, overdistention and detrusor atony. There is mild-to-moderate trabeculation. The external sphincter is flaccid, and so there is no interruption of flow. Voiding may be fairly efficient with abdominal pressure. This type of bladder generally is characterized by a large capacity, no involuntary detrusor contractions, low intravesical pressure, and mild trabeculation.

Treatment of suprasacral lesions generally consists of conservative methods initially, in order to attempt to improve bladder emptying. These consist of catheter drainage during the period of "spinal shock," either continuous or intermittent, followed by bladder training using "trigger areas," crede, timed double and triple voiding. Transurethral resection of the bladder neck or sphincter can be tried to decrease resistance to flow. Pudendal block, neurectomy, anterior rhizotomy are other methods of management.

CASE 57: 74-YEAR-OLD MALE WITH CEREBROVASCULAR ACCIDENT

HISTORY

A 74-year-old man having suffered a recent cerebrovascular accident was brought to the emergency room. He had lost consciousness momentarily, then awoke with slurred speech, and inability to move his right arm and leg. There was a history of adult onset diabetes mellitus controlled by diet alone. There was no history of myocardial infarction. He had had nocturia two times nightly, with some decrease in force and caliber of the urinary stream, but had not other urinary symptoms.

PHYSICAL EXAMINATION

The patient was markedly disoriented and dysarthric. There was a right flaccid hemiplegia. The right extremities were markedly weak. Deep tendon reflexes were hyperactive more on the right than the left. There was a right side positive Babinski sign. The bladder was seen to be distended three finger breadths above the symphysis pubis. On rectal examination, the prostate was only slightly enlarged and benign. The remainder of the examination was within normal limits.

LABORATORY DATA

Complete blood count was normal. Blood urea nitrogen 17mg%. Blood sugar on admission 174mg%.

A catheter was inserted and 700cc urine obtained, which was normal on routine and microscopic examination, and showed no growth on culture. Remainder of a chemical profile (SMA 12) was all within normal limits.

CLINICAL COURSE

The patient was admitted to the hospital, and given the routine supportive care for his vascular accident. He was placed on intermittent catheterization every four to six hours because he was unable to void. His sensorium and speech gradually improved, and within a week, he was beginning to speak intelligibly. On the fifth hospital day, he began to void spontaneously, and his residual urine fell to less than 75cc. He had frequency of urination, as well as urgency, to the point where he frequently wet his bed or pajamas. An intravenous urogram was performed, which showed normal upper urinary tracts and a fairly smooth bladder. Cystometry and integrated sphincter electromyography performed ten days after admission revealed detrusor hyperflexia with detrusor-sphincter dyssynergia (Fig. 57.1). Cystoscopy showed only mild trabeculation and a partially obstructing prostate gland.

As his sensorium improved, he was better able to control his incontinence, but continued to have frequency of urination. His residual urine remained in the range of 30-40cc without drugs, and he was discharged voiding well, but with mild frequency and nocturia every 3 hours.

QUESTIONS

1. The voiding dysfunction in this patient is secondary to interruption of which of the pathways of bladder innervation?
   A. Pudendal nucleus
   B. Reticulospinal tracts
   C. Frontal cortex to reticular formation in brain stem
   D. Cerebellar-reticular formation connections

2. The initial episode of urinary retention in this patient is secondary to:
   A. Benign enlargement of the prostate
   B. Detrusor-sphincter dyssynergia
   C. Rachischisis or spinal shock
   D. Incompetent bladder neck
   E. Spasm of external sphincter

3. Which of the following pharmacologic agents might be of beneficial value in this patient?
   A. Bethanechol
   B. Ephedrine
   C. Propanalol
   D. Phenoxybenzamine
   E. Dantrolene

4. Interpretation of the results of cystometry are dependent on which of the following factors?
   A. Symptom complaint
   B. Results of the general physical, urologic and neurologic examination
   C. Presence or absence of detrusor reflex on cystometrogram
   D. Description of sensory changes during cystometry
   E. All of the above

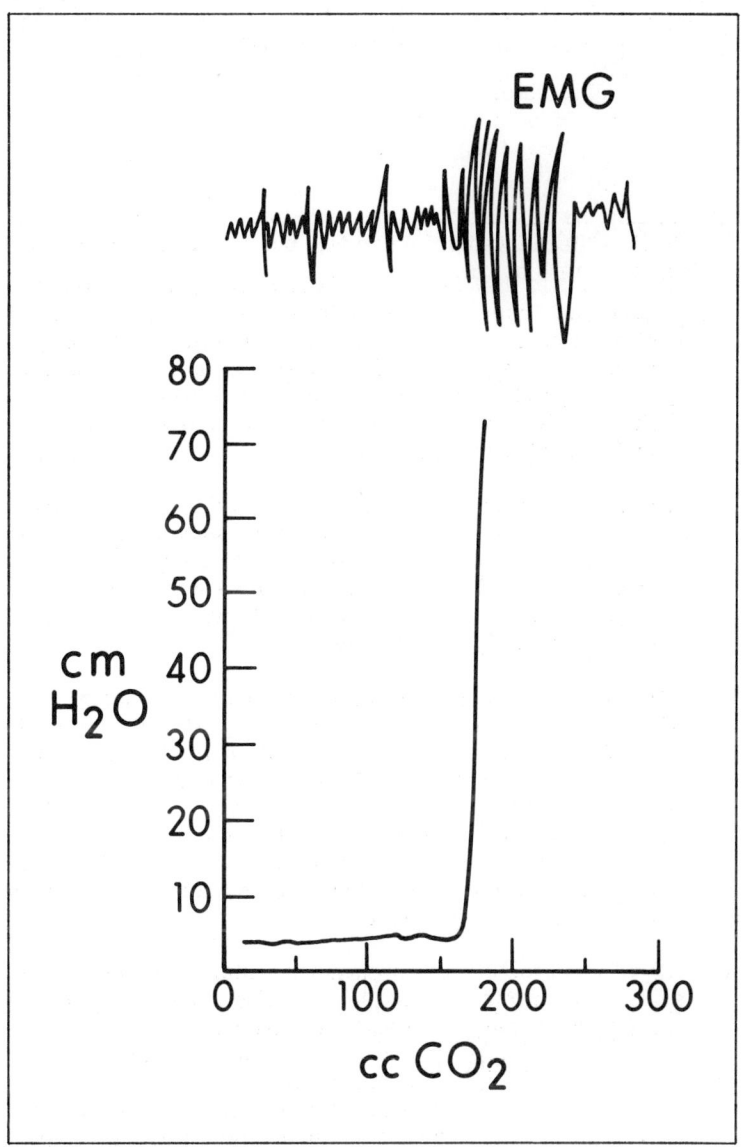

FIG. 57.1: Cystometrogram and integrated sphincter electromyography showing detrusor hyperflexia and detrusor-sphincter dyssynergia.

Case 57 — Neurogenic Bladder

5. All of the neurologic conditions below are associated with interruption of loop I pathways of Bradley, except:
   A. Stroke
   B. Brain tumor
   C. Parkinson's disease
   D. Spinal cord tumor
   E. Dementia

ANSWERS AND DISCUSSION

1. (C) Loop I in the classification of Bradley consists of pathways to and from the frontal lobes to the pontine-mesenphalic reticular formation in the brain stem. Neurologic lesions of any sort that affect these cortical and subcortical areas produce partial or complete release of the micturition reflex from volitional control, thus causing a detrusor hyperflexic bladder and a small bladder capacity.

2. (C) The initial episode of shock associated with the acute onset of the cerebrovascular accident can be associated with detrusor areflexia, with inability to void, or a very large residual urine. This usually lasts only several days. Then the hyperflexia takes over, causing the usual frequency, urgency and urgency incontinence.

3. (E) Dantrolene is a skeletal muscle relaxant, and may be of some benefit in relaxing a markedly spastic external sphincter. This was not the situation in this case, and therefore it was not used. This patient was able to void without the use of any pharmacological agents. The other agents given as choices have no effect on skeletal muscle. Since the patient was able to void with only a small residual, agents affecting the detrusor or smooth muscle sphincter were not employed here.

4. (E) The cystometrogram cannot be interpreted in and of itself. The patient's symptoms must be evaluated. Is there frequency, urgency, urgency incontinence, etc.? This would be seen in the presence of detrusor hyperreflexia. Is there difficulty in initiating the stream? In this case, cystometry would reveal detrusor areflexia. Of course, the general physical, urologic and neurologic findings must be brought into the total evaluation of the patient. The description of sensory changes during filling must be noted and recorded on the cystometric chart.

5. (D) Loop I consists of pathways from the frontal lobes to the pontine-mesencephalic reticular formation. This would not be affected by a spinal cord lesion. All of the others are diseases affecting the cerebral area, and are associated with interruption of these pathways.

REFERENCES

1. Bradley WE, Timm GW, and Scott FB: Cystometry I, Introduction. Urology, Vol. V, Mar. 1975, p. 578.

2. Bradley WE, Timm GW, and Scott FB: Innervation of the detrusor muscle and urethra. Urol Clin of N Amer, Vol. 1, No. 1, Feb. 1974, p. 3.

CASE 58: 17-YEAR-OLD BOY WITH NECK INJURY

HISTORY

A 17-year-old boy was admitted to the hospital with a neck injury sustained by diving into a pool and striking his head at the bottom. When he was pulled from the pool, he was unable to move his arms and legs.

PHYSICAL EXAMINATION

Blood pressure and pulse were normal. There was an evident quadriparesis with a sensory level to C5, and there was spastic quadriplegia. The bladder was distended almost to the umbilicus. The remainder of the physical examination was within normal limits.

LABORATORY DATA

CBC, urinalysis, chemical profile, EKG and chest x-ray all within normal limits. X-rays of the cervical spine revealed a fracture of C5 and C6.

CLINICAL COURSE

The patient was admitted to the neurosurgical service, and underwent laminectomy in the areas of the fracture. His quadriplegia remained complete, however, and showed no response to decompression. He was treated on the rehabilitation service, as well as urologically, with intermittent catheterization. After 7 weeks on intermittent catheterization, he began to void spontaneously. He was also incontinent at this time, and was placed on a condom catheter. Cystometrogram and integrated sphincter electromyography revealed a hypertonic bladder with involuntary contractions and detrusor-sphincter dyssynergia. A urethral pressure profile showed a very high urethral resistance in the area of the external sphincter (Fig. 58.1).

A residual urine at this time was 150cc with a bladder capacity of 350cc. He underwent sphincterotomy. Following this, he continued to be intermittently incontinent, but could void with a better stream, and showed only 50-75cc residual urine. His upper tracts are normal on intravenous urogram. A retrograde cystogram shows no evidence of reflux, and the bladder shows marked trabeculation. His urine remains sterile on suppressive therapy with Mandelamine.

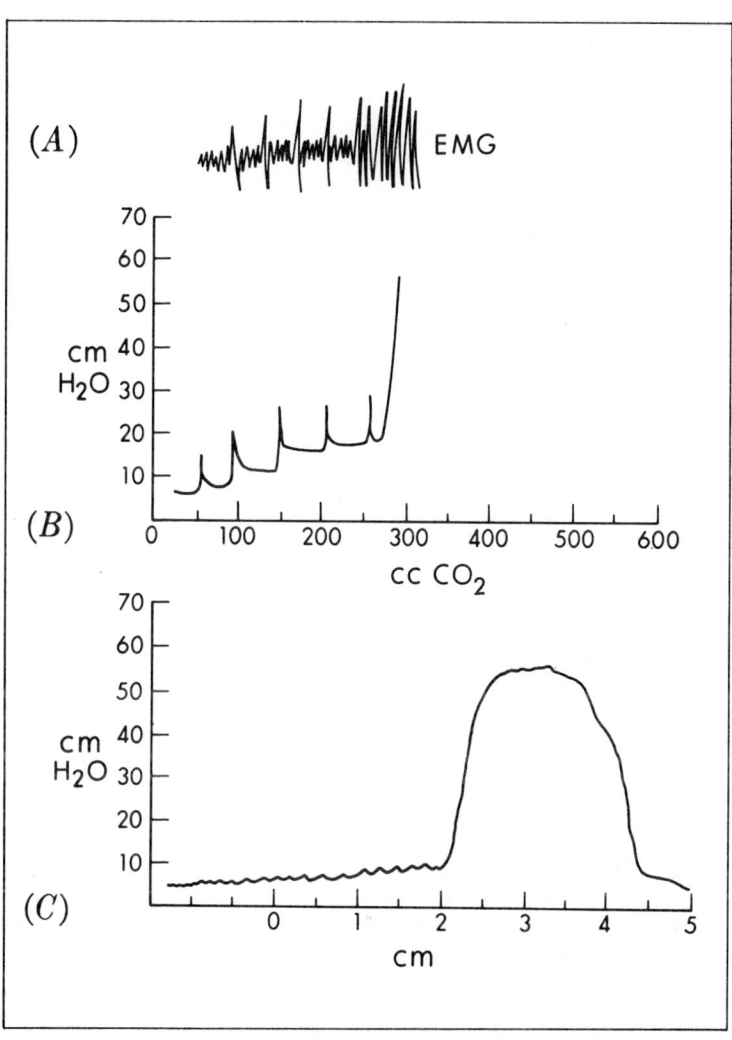

FIG. 58.1: (A) Integrated electromyography showing sphincter dyssynergia; (B) Cystometrogram with involuntary contractions and detrusor hyperflexia; (C) Urethral pressure profile.

QUESTIONS

1. All of the neurologic findings below are associated with suprasacral cord lesions, except:
   A. Frequent upper tract deterioration
   B. Uninhibited bladder contraction
   C. Spasticity of external sphincter
   D. Decreased bladder capacity
   E. Absence of bulbocavernous reflex

2. Which of the following are frequently helpful in attaining bladder emptying in suprasacral cord lesions?
   A. Bethanechol
   B. Ephedrine
   C. Sphincterotomy
   D. Pro-Banthine
   E. A & C

3. In the acutely injured spinal cord patient, the initial phase of urologic management is best handled by:
   A. Foley catheter drainage with intermittent irrigation
   B. Three-way Foley catheter with continuous bladder irrigation
   C. Intermittent catheterization
   D. Suprapubic cystotomy
   E. Allow the patient to void spontaneously, since he will probably empty the bladder well

4. Detrusor sphincter dyssynergia is indicative of:
   A. Relaxation of the sphincter at the time of bladder contraction
   B. Increased activity of the sphincter at the time of bladder contraction
   C. Relaxation of the urethral sphincter with concomitant relaxation of the detrusor
   D. Contraction of the sphincter with relaxation of the detrusor
   E. All of the above

5. Which of the following pharmacologic agents would be useful in the treatment of detrusor hyperflexia?
   A. Isoproterenol
   B. Bethanechol chloride
   C. Phenoxybenzamine
   D. Propanolol
   E. Pro-Banthine (Propanthaline)

Neurogenic Bladder

6. Autonomic dysreflexia is characterized by all of the following, except:
   A. Excessive sweating
   B. Occipital headache
   C. Facial flushing
   D. Nausea
   E. Hypotension

7. Autonomic dysreflexia occurs in complete spinal cord injury above the level of:
   A. Sacral segments 2 and 3
   B. Lumbar 5
   C. Lumbar 1
   D. Thoracic 7
   E. Cervical 6

ANSWERS AND DISCUSSION

1. (E) With lesions in the suprasacral area, the cord below the lesion frequently becomes hyperirritable, causing severe effects on the bladder. Uninhibited contractions frequently occur, and there is a hyperflexic bladder with spasticity of the external sphincter. Hypertrophy of the detrusor develops, and, frequently, reflux occurs. All this contributes to upper urinary tract deterioration. In suprasacral lesions, the bulbocavernous reflex remains intact.

2. (C) As previously stated, in suprasacral lesions, the external sphincter and perineal muscles become spastic, causing increased resistance to flow and residual urine. Cutting the sphincter muscle transurethrally can cause a decrease in the resistance to flow with more efficient voiding. This, of course, must be done with care, with, perhaps, measurements made of urethral pressure profiles during the course of the procedure in the hope of not causing complete urinary incontinence.

3. (C) Spinal shock, with the invariable accompaniment of detrusor areflexia, is best managed by intermittent catheterization. There is a lower incidence of infection with this method, and allowing the bladder to fill and empty with physiologic volumes maintains some degree of normality to voiding. Continuous Foley catheter drainage, with or without irrigation, will lead to a higher incidence of more severe infections.

4. (B) Normally, the external sphincter of the urethra should relax synchronously with detrusor contraction. In detrusor-

sphincter dyssynergia, the sphincter shows increased activity at the time of detrusor contraction, causing increased resistance to the flow of urine and inefficient voiding.

5. (E) Propanthalene (Pro-Banthine) is a parasympatholytic agent used to relax detrusor activity, and is frequently used in the treatment of detrusor hyperflexia.

6. (E) Hypertensive crises may occur with autonomic dysreflexia in lesions of the upper thoracic and cervical cord. They are also characterized by excessive sweating, occipital headaches, facial flushing, nausea, as well as chills. They are initiated by a full bladder, and characteristically occur just prior to voiding.

7. E

REFERENCES

1. O'Flynn JD: Neurogenic bladder in spinal cord injury. Urol Clin N Amer I:155, 1974.

2. McGuire EJ, Wagner GM, and Weiss R: Treatment of autonomic dysreflexia with phenoxybenzamine. J Urol 115:53, 1976.

CASE 59: 48-YEAR-OLD MALE WITH FRACTURE OF L4 AND L5 VERTEBRAE AND URINARY TRACT INFECTION

HISTORY

A 48-year-old male was seen in consultation because of a urinary tract infection and fever. He had been admitted to the neurosurgical service 6 weeks previously because of a fracture to L4 and L5 vertebral bodies, sustained in a fall from a scaffold. These were operated on, and pins were placed in the vertebra for stabilization. Following the injury, he was paraplegic and had been on rehabilitation medicine. Because he was unable to void at all, a Foley had been left indwelling for the past 6 weeks, and changed at weekly intervals. He complained of pain in the left testicle.

PHYSICAL EXAMINATION

Temp 103°. Pulse 120 regular. Blood pressure 120/80. There was complete paralysis of both lower extremities with a sensory level to L4. A Foley catheter was in place. The left hemiscrotum was markedly swollen, reddened and exquisitely tender. There was an area of fluctuance in the anterior portion of the scrotum. The prostate was normal in size and consistency. The remainder of the physical examination was within normal limits.

LABORATORY DATA

Urinalysis showed innumerable WBC and RBC and many bacteria. Urine culture grew Proteus species, greater than 100,000 organisms per ml. Blood urea nitrogen, creatinine were within normal limits. CBC and SMA were normal. An intravenous urogram at this time showed normal upper tracts, with no evidence of calculi or obstruction.

CLINICAL COURSE

A percutaneous cystostomy was immediately performed, and the Foley catheter removed. The patient was placed on gentamycin intramuscularly, and Keflin intravenously. His temperature gradually fell, and the scrotal mass and tenderness improved until only a small nodule could be felt in the left epididymis. Cystometrogram with integrated sphincter electromyography was performed, which showed detrusor areflexia, as well as normal sphincter activity, but no sphincter relaxation with straining (Fig. 59.1). Because of the urethritis and epididymitis, it was elected to perform a continent vesicostomy in this patient (Fig. 59.2).

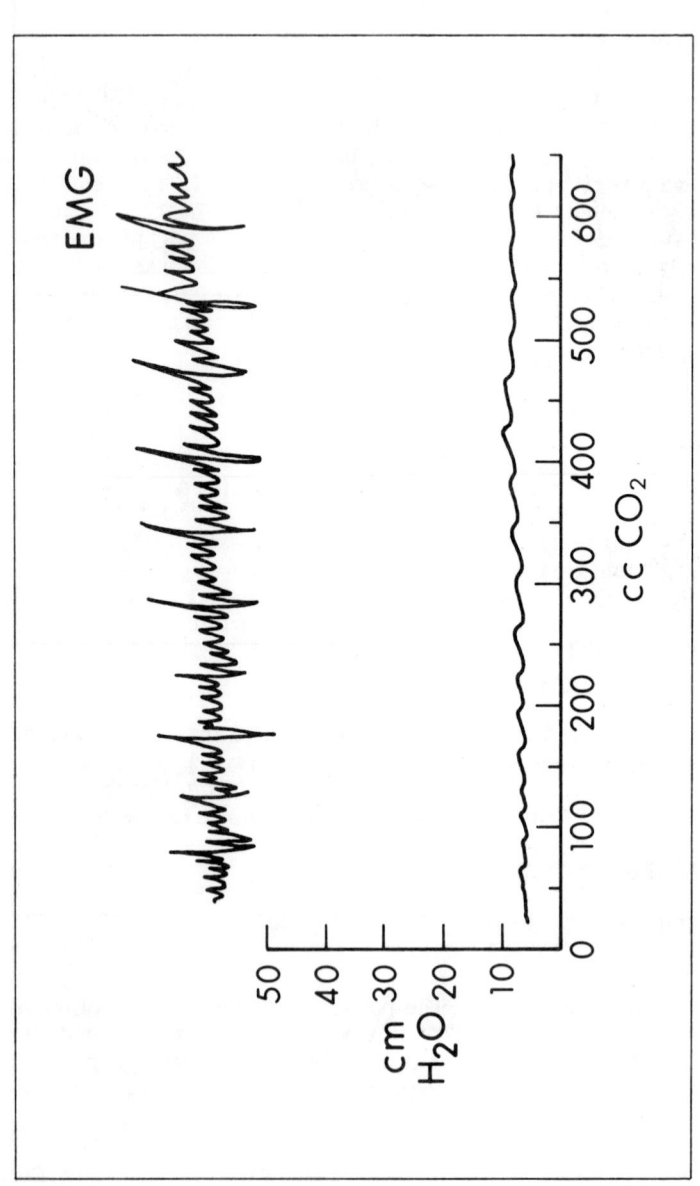

FIG. 59.1: Cystometrogram and integrated sphincter electromyography showing detrusor areflexia.

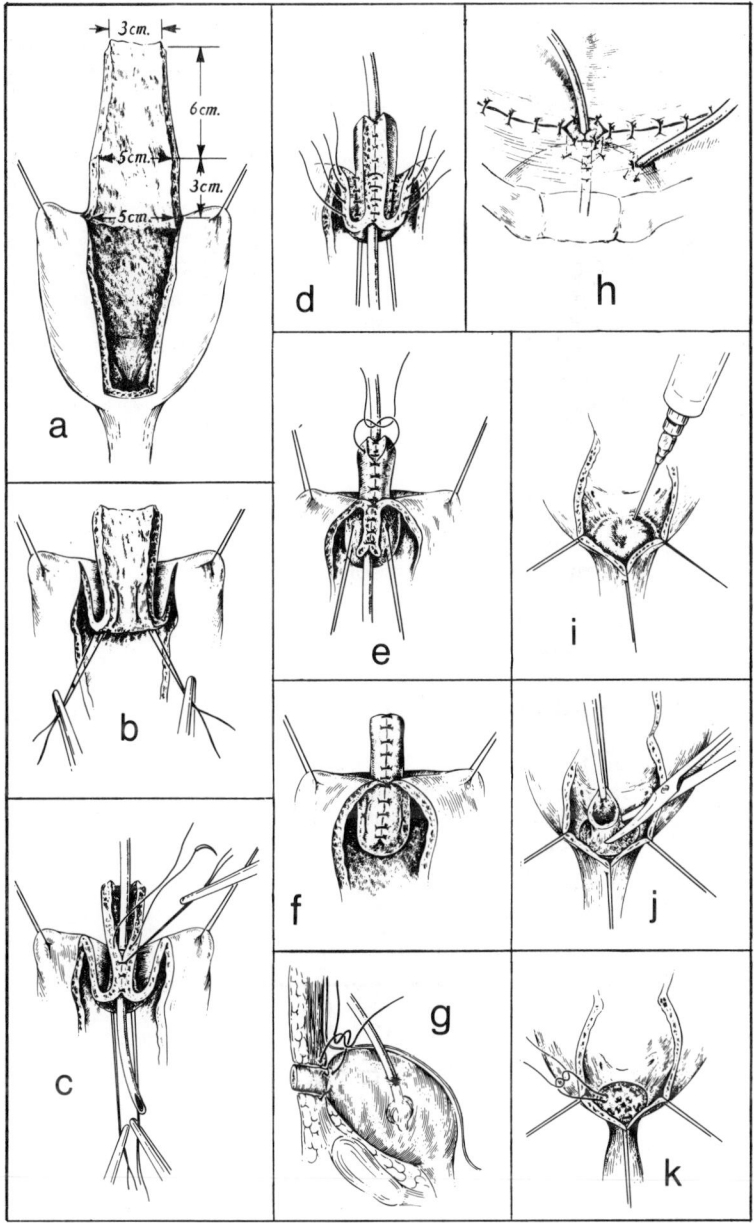

FIG. 59.2: Steps in performance of a continent vesicostomy.

292/ Case 59　　　　　　　　　　　　　　　Neurogenic Bladder

This was performed in February, 1974. He tolerated the procedure well, and continues to catheterize himself through the vesicostomy. His cystometrogram continues to show detrusor areflexia, and he is unable to void per urethra. Six months after his continent vesicostomy, he developed right renal colic, and underwent right ureterolithotomy for a large stone. To date, his I.V. urogram and cystogram remain normal, as is his BUN and creatinine.

QUESTIONS

1. All of the following are characteristic of bladder dysfunction secondary to a lesion of the sacral cord, except:
   A. Low intravesical pressure
   B. Large capacity bladder
   C. Involuntary detrusor contractions
   D. Decreased sphincter tone
   E. Bladder trabeculation

2. Recovery from spinal shock can be determined by:
   A. Cystometer studies
   B. Return of sensation in some areas
   C. Return of reflex activity
   D. The "ice water test"
   E. All of the above

3. The characteristic cystometrogram in sacral lesions would show:
   A. Bladder capacity of less than 300cc
   B. Bladder capacity of more than 500cc
   C. A strong detrusor contraction
   D. Numerous involuntary detrusor contractions
   E. None of the above

4. Alpha adrenergic stimulation:
   A. Decreases outlet resistance
   B. Increases intraurethral pressure
   C. Is produced by phenoxybenzamine
   D. Is produced by ephedrine
   E. Produces relaxation of the detrusor

5. Which of the following are helpful in the treatment of neurogenic bladder secondary to a sacral lesion?
   A. Sphincterotomy
   B. Ephedrine
   C. Phenoxybenzamine
   D. Transurethral resection
   E. None of the above

Neurogenic Bladder

ANSWERS AND DISCUSSION

1. (C) The characteristic cystometrogram seen in sacral cord lesions is that of a perfectly flat curve, with no evidence of involuntary bladder contractions. There is generally a large bladder capacity with evidence of trabeculation, as well as poor sphincter tone present. The intravesical pressure remains low during bladder filling.

2. (E) Spinal shock after an injury may last from weeks to months. If there is a suprasacral injury, there may be return of reflex activity in the lower extremities. Spontaneous voiding may occur around the catheter. The cystometric curve may show a "shift to the left," i.e., a smaller bladder capacity with some return, albeit small, of detrusor contractions. Anal sphincter tone and bulbocavernous reflexes may return in suprasacral lesions. By instilling 9 ml of saline solution at 3°C, a straight catheter is forcefully ejected. This is known as a positive "ice water test," and signifies some return of function.

3. (B) The usual cystometric findings with a sacral lesion would show a bladder capacity above normal levels (600-1,000cc or more), decreased intravesical pressure, and the absence of uninhibited contractions. There are hypoactive peripheral reflexes and flaccid muscle tone. On removal of the catheter, voiding does not usually occur.

4. (D) Ephedrine is an alpha-adrenergic stimulator, and will cause contraction of the smooth muscle sphincter at the vesical neck. It may result in an increase in urethral pressure (B), but this is not invariably the case.

5. (E) Transurethral resection of the vesical neck and prostate may sometimes be useful, but when the main problem is an inability to produce a detrusor contraction to empty the bladder, this will often fail. TUR combined with Crede may work in some cases.

REFERENCE

1. Schneider KM, Reid RE, and Fruchtman B: Continent vesicostomy - surgical technique. Urology 6:740, Dec., 1975.

CASE 60: 34-YEAR-OLD MALE WITH DIFFICULTY VOIDING

HISTORY

A 34-year-old salesman was seen because of difficulty voiding and a recent urinary tract infection. He stated that he had to sit to void all his life and had to strain very hard in order to complete voiding; he never felt that he emptied his bladder completely. He had recently been admitted to another hospital for a urinary tract infection with fever to 105° and treated with ampicillin with prompt response of the infection. He continued to have marked difficulty in voiding. He stated that at birth he had "surgery on his lower spine" but was not aware of its exact nature.

PHYSICAL EXAMINATION

Blood pressure and pulse normal. Urologic examination was entirely within normal limits. The bulbocavernous reflex, however, was absent. There was a well-healed longitudinal scar on the back over the lumbosacral region.

QUESTIONS

1. The primary diagnosis at this time would be:
   A. Congenital myelomeningocele with neurogenic bladder
   B. Non-neurogenic neurogenic bladder
   C. Psychoneurosis
   D. Diabetes mellitus with hypotonic bladder
   E. None of the above

LABORATORY DATA

CBC, normal. Urinalysis at this time was normal. Urine culture and sensitivity showed no growth. A plain film of the abdomen showed a spina bifida of L5, S1, S2 and S3. Intravenous urogram revealed normal upper urinary tracts. The bladder was moderately trabeculated; there was a large postvoid residual urine.

CLINICAL COURSE

Cystometrogram with integrated sphincter electromyography was performed which revealed a markedly hypotonic bladder with a capacity of 600cc, and a poor detrusor contraction which only generated 30cm of H_2O pressure. The sphincter relaxed normally at this time (Fig. 60.1A&B). Urine flowmetry revealed a very slow stream with an average flow of less than 5cc/sec and a maximum flow rate of 7cc/sec (Fig. 60.1). Cystoscopy was normal with no evidence of mechanical obstruction.

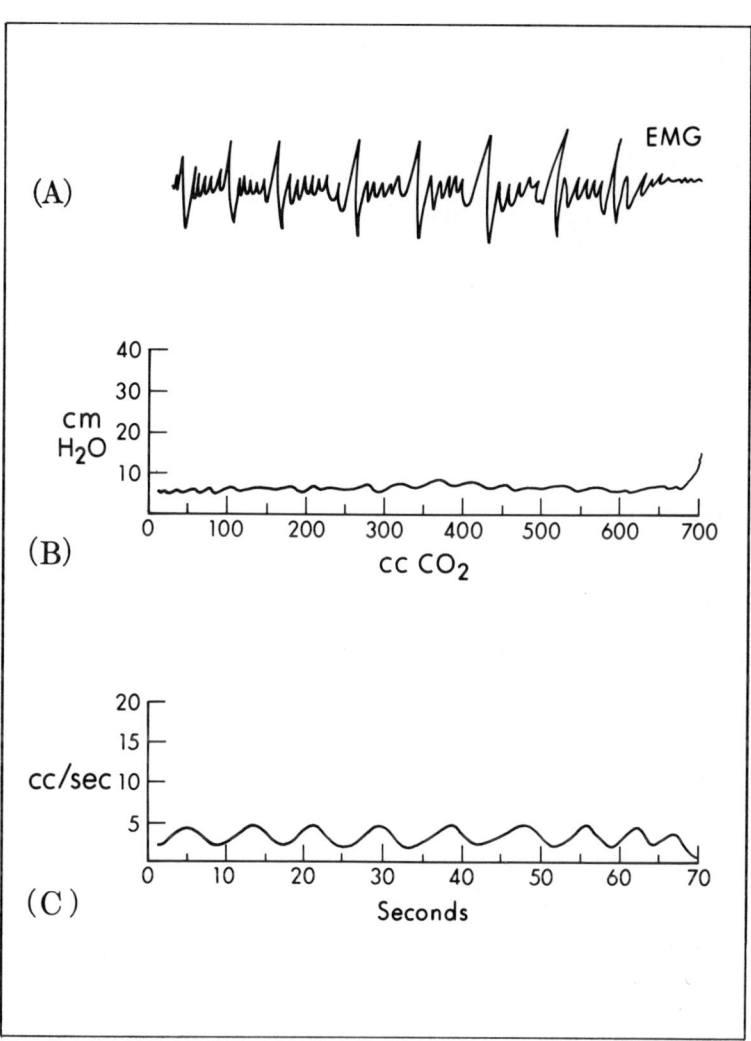

FIG. 60.1: (A) Integrated sphincter electromyography. (B) Cystometrogram with detrusor hyporeflexia. (C) Urine flowmetry.

296/ Case 60   Neurogenic Bladder

2. The normal urine flow for a 34-year-old male should be:
    A. 20cc/sec
    B. 25cc/sec
    C. 15cc/sec
    D. 35cc/sec
    E. Over 40cc/sec

3. Pharmacologic agents that may be useful in this patient are:
    A. Bethanechol
    B. Oxybutynin
    C. Phenoxybenzamine
    D. Propantheline
    E. A & C

He was placed on bethanechol 25mg four times daily, and within a short period of time, he was voiding better. He was completely elated, since it was the first time in his life that he could stand at the urinal to void. A repeat study was performed which showed a normal cystometric curve, normal sphincter EMG. Urine flowmetry showed an increase in flow to an average of 14cc/sec, and a maximum flow rate of 18cc/sec. More importantly, he was able to empty his bladder without residual urine (Fig. 60.2). He continues to do well on the above dose of bethanechol.

(T)RUE OR (F)ALSE:

4. Filling of the bladder is said to be related to sympathetic innervation, and emptying to parasympathetic.

5. All of the following drugs cause increased outlet resistance, except:
    A. Ephedrine sulfate
    B. Phenylephrine
    C. Imipramine
    D. Phentolamine
    E. Phenylpropanolamine

6. All of the following drugs will cause decreased bladder contractility except:
    A. Atropine
    B. Propantheline
    C. Oxybutynin
    D. Acetylcholine
    E. Imipramine

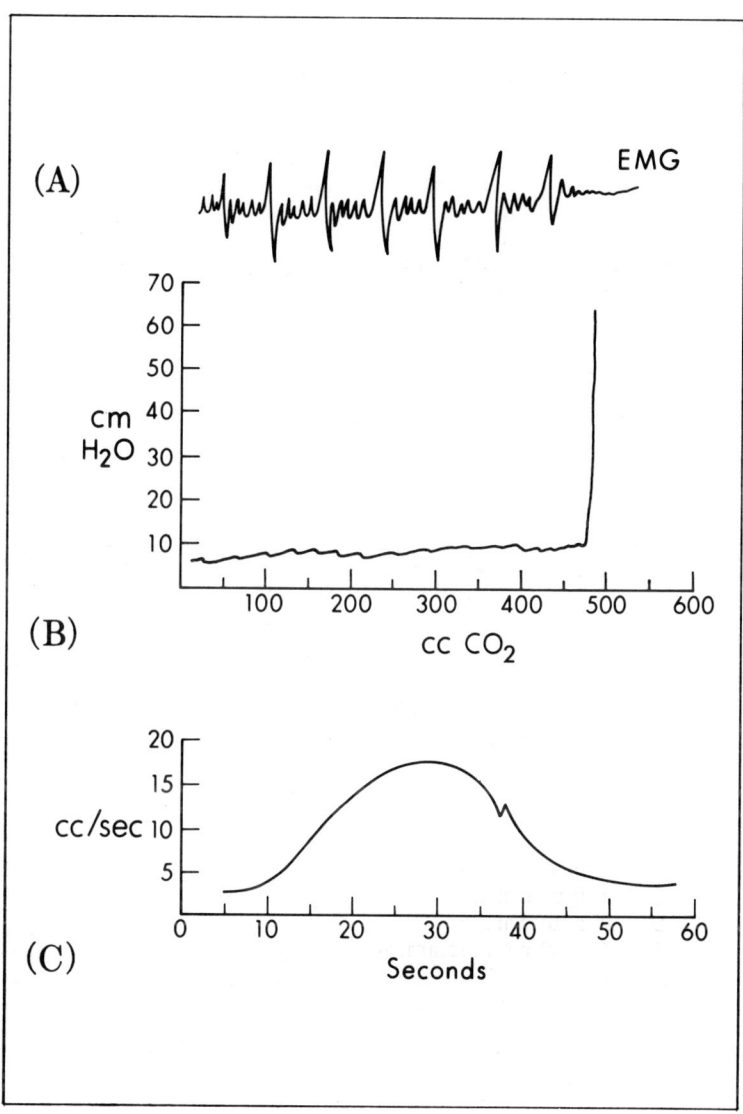

FIG. 60.2: (A) Sphincter electromyography. (B) Cystometrogram. (C) Urine flowmetry after 3 months of bethanechol 25 mg q.i.d.

ANSWERS AND DISCUSSION

1. (A) Congenital myelomeningocele that involves only the cauda equina can present in adulthood with only urinary symptoms, as in this case. This was apparently glanced over or missed at his previous admission to another hospital. Because there were no somatic nerves involved, only S2, S3 and S4, there were no peripheral neurologic signs to be found.

2. (B) The normal flow rate for a young male should be about 25cc/sec. Female flow rates are somewhat higher.

3. (E) Bethanechol, a parasympathomimetic, would be useful here in order to attain more efficient voiding to empty the bladder. If this fails to achieve emptying, phenoxybenzamine could be added. This is an alpha-adrenergic blocking agent, which would cause relaxation of the smooth muscle sphincter to decrease resistance of the bladder neck.

4. (T) The body of the bladder is primarily innervated with beta-adrenergic fibers, and the base by alpha-adrenergic sympathetic fibers. Stimulation of the former cause bladder relaxation, and allows for filling. At the same time, alpha-adrenergic stimulation causes contraction of the muscle around the bladder neck maintaining continence. Emptying is due to parasympathetic stimulation causing contraction of the detrusor muscle.

5. (D) Phentolamine is an alpha-adrenergic blocking agent, and, therefore, will cause decreased outlet resistance. The rest of the drugs mentioned are alpha-adrenergic stimulators, and will cause increased bladder outlet resistance.

6. (D) Acetylcholine is a parasympathomimetic, and will cause an increase in intravesical contractility. The other agents are parasympathetic depressants, and will cause a decrease in bladder contractility.

REFERENCE

1. Khanna OP: Disorder of micturition: Neuropharmacologic basis and results of drug therapy. Urology 8:316, Oct. 1976.

DIAGNOSES: CASE STUDIES

URINARY OBSTRUCTION (Cases 1-8)

1: Posterior Urethral Valves
2: Bladder Neck Contracture with Bladder Diverticulum
3: Benign Prostate Hypertrophy
4: Ectopic Ureterocele
5: Double Collecting System with Obstruction of Upper Segment
6: Ureteropelvic Junction Obstruction
7: Ureteropelvic Junction Obstruction
8: Urethral Stricture

URINARY INJURY (Cases 9-17)

9: Renal Laceration - Closed Injury
10: Renal Laceration - Stab Wound
11: Ureteral Avulsion
12: Ureterovaginal Fistula
13: Ruptured Bladder - Closed Injury
14: Ruptured Bladder - Open Injury
15: Rupture of Distal Urethra
16: Rupture of Membranous Urethra
17: Vesicovaginal Fistula

VESICOURETERAL REFLUX (Cases 18-21)

18: Vesicoureteral Reflux, Conservative Treatment
19: Vesicoureteral Reflux (2^O to Valves)
20: Vesicoureteral Reflux
21: Vesicoureteral Reflux Complication of Bladder Surgery

"NONSPECIFIC" INFECTIONS (Cases 22-26)

22: Chronic Pyelonephritis; Contracted Kidneys
23: Renal Carbuncle
24: Perinephric Abscess
25: Papillary Necrosis
26: Cystitis 2^O Adjacent Inflammatory Disease

TUBERCULOSIS (Cases 27-29)

RENAL TUMORS (Cases 30-39)

- 30: Renal Cell Carcinoma
- 31: Transitional Cell Carcinoma of the Renal Pelvis
- 32: Transitional Cell Carcinoma of Ureter
- 33: Angiomyolipoma
- 34: Renal Cell Carcinoma with Solitary Pulmonary "Metastasis"
- 35: Wilms' Tumor
- 36: Simple Renal Cyst
- 37: Multicystistic Kidney
- 38: Polycystic Kidney
- 39: Peripelvic Cyst

BLADDER TUMORS (Cases 40-43)

- 40: Bladder Papillomas
- 41: Bladder Tumor (TURBT)
- 42: Bladder Tumor, Segmental Resection
- 43: Bladder Tumor: Preoperative Radiotherapy and Radical Cystectomy

CARCINOMA OF THE PROSTATE (Cases 44-46)

- 44: Carcinoma of Prostate, Stage A
- 45: Carcinoma of Prostate, Stage B
- 46: Carcinoma of Prostate, Stage B

RENAL CALCULI (Cases 47-53)

- 47: Ureteral Calculus
- 48: Renal Pelvic Calculus
- 49: Radiolucent Calculus
- 50: Staghorn Calculus
- 51: Bilateral Staghorn Calculus
- 52: Bladder Calculi
- 53: Urethral Calculus in Diverticulum

THE ADRENAL GLAND (Cases 54-56)

- 54: Cushing's Syndrome
- 55: Pheochromocytoma
- 56: Pheochromocytoma

NEUROGENIC BLADDER (Cases 57-60)

57: Detrusor Hyperflexia Secondary to Cerebrovascular Accident
58: Detrusor Hyperflexia Secondary to Spinal Cord Injury C5 and C6
59: Detrusor Areflexia Due to Trauma at L5
60: Detrusor Hyporeflexia Secondary to Myelomeningocele

INDEX and POST-TEST

INDEX

Acetylcholine, 298
Adenocarcinoma, Kidney, 146-147
Adenoma, Kidney, 146
Adrenal Gland, 264-276
  Anatomy, 264
  Embryology, 264
Allopurinal, 225
Angioma, Kidney, 146
Anterior Rhizotomy, 278
Autonomic Dysreflexia, 288

Benign Prostatic Hyperplasia, 1, 13-16
Benzidine, 199
Bethanochol, 298
Bladder
  Calculi, 254-257
  Diverticulum, 9-12
  Emptying of, 277
  "Herald Lesion" of, 129-131
  Injuries, 46
  Neoplasm, 199-212
    Classification, 199-200
    Etiology, 199
    Treatment, 200
      Cystectomy, 209-212
      Segmental Resection, 207-208
      TUR, 201-206
  Neurogenic, 277-298
    Cerebrovascular Accident and, 279-283
    Classification, 277
    Fracture Vertebra and, 287-293
    Myelomeningocele and, 294-298
    Quadriplegia and, 284-288
  Treatment of, 278
  Rupture
    Intraperitoneal, 71-73
    Extraperitoneal, 74-77
  Uninhibited Contractions of, 287

Calcium Oxalate Stones, 224
Calculi
  Bladder, 254-257
  Renal, 224-225
Carbuncle, Renal, 116-119
Chronic Pyelonephritis, 112-115
Continent Vesicostomy, 291
Cushing's Syndrome, 264-268
Cyst, Renal (see Renal, cysts)
Cystine, 224-225
Cystometrogram, 282-293

Dantrolene, 282
Detrusor-Sphincter Dyssynergia, 287-288
Diversion, Urinary, 7
Diverticulitis, 129
Diverticulum
  Bladder, 1-2, 9-12
  Urethral, 258-263
Double Collecting System, 23-26

Ephedrine, 293
Epididymitis, 111
Estrogens, 213

Fibroma, Renal, 146
Fistula
  Cutaneous, 144
  Ureteroperineal, 83-88
  Ureterovaginal, 64-70
  Vesicovaginal, 89-92
    Repair of, 90

Ganglioneuroma, Adrenal, 264
Gunshot Wound, 77

Hydronephrosis, 4
Hyperparathyroidism, 224
Hypervitaminosis D, 225

Idiopathic Hypercalcuria, 224-225
Infection
  Chronic Pyelonephritis, 112-115
  "Nonspecific", 111
  Perinephric Abscess, 120-124
Injury
  Bladder, 46, 71-77
  Renal, 45-46, 48-58
  Ureteral, 46, 59-70
  Urethral, 47, 78-88
Interlocking Sounds, 47

Kidney (see Renal)

Latzko Operation, 90
Leadbetter-Politano Ureteroneocystostomy, 100
Lipoma, Kidney, 146

Magnesium Oxide, 225
Multicystic Kidney (see Renal, cysts)
Myelomeningocele, 298
Myoma, 146

Naphthylamine, 199
Nephroureterectomy, 155, 160

Obstruction, Urinary, 1
  Pathophysiology of, 1-2
  Ureteropelvic Junction, 27-39
Orchiectomy, 213

Papillary Necrosis, 125-128
Perinephric Abscess, 120-124
Peripelvic Cyst, 146
Phentolamine, 298
Pheochromocytoma, 269-276
Polycystic Kidney (see Renal, cysts)
Presacral CO_2 Insufflation, 265
Progestagens, 213
Propantheline, 296
Prostate
  Benign Hyperplasia, 13-16
  Carcinoma, 15, 213, 223
    Classification, 215
    Radical Prostatectomy for, 217-219
    Radiotherapy for, 220-223
Prostatitis, 111
Pudental Nerve Block, 278
Pyelogenic Cyst, 146
Pyeloplasty, 27, 32, 35

Radiotherapy
  Bladder Tumors, 212
  Prostate Tumors, 213
Reflux, Vesicoureteral, 93-110
Renal
  Calculi, 224-225
    Pyelolithotomy for, 226-228, 236-239
    Staghorn, 240-253
    Ureterolithotomy for, 229-235
    Uric Acid, 236-239
  Cysts, 146
    Multicystic Kidney, 189-190
    Parapelvic, 193
    Polycystic, 146, 191-192
    Solitary, 184-188
  Duplication, 23-26
  Dysplasia, 197
  Infection, 111-115
  Injury, 45-46
    Laceration, 48-58

Neoplasm
  Benign, 146
    Angiomyolipoma, 166-169
    Malignant, 146-148
      Adenocarcinoma, 150-154, 170-177
      Transitional Cell Carcinoma, 155-160
      Wilms' Tumor, 178-183
  Obstruction, 1-44
  Papillary Necrosis, 125-128
  Tubular Acidosis, 225

Segmental Resection, Bladder (see Bladder, neoplasm)
Sphincterotomy, 284, 287
Spina Bifida, 277
Spinal Cord Lesions, 277
Spinal Shock, 287
Squamous Cell Carcinoma, 199
Stricture, Urethral, 1
Sympathicoblastoma, 264

Thio-Tepa, 200-201, 204
Transitional Cell Carcinoma
  Bladder, 199
  Kidney, 146-147, 155-160
  Ureter, 161-165
Transurethral Resection
  Bladder Tumor, 200
  Prostate, 16
Tryptophane, 199
Tuberculosis, 132-133
  Generalized, 144-145
  Renal, 138-143
  Ureteral, 134-137
Tumors
  Bladder, 199-212
  Kidney
    Benign, 146, 166-169
    Malignant, 146-148, 150-160, 170-183

Prostate, 15, 213, 223

Ureter
  Injury, 46
    Blunt, 59-63
    Postsurgical, 64-70, 83-88, 89-92
  Neoplasm, 161-165
  Reimplantation, 100, 101
Ureteral Orifice, Ectopic, 26
Ureterocele, Ectopic, 17-22
Ureteroneocystostomy, 65
Ureteropelvic Junction Obstruction, 27-39
Urethra
  Diverticulum, 258-263
  Injuries, 47, 78-82
  Stricture, 40-44
Uric Acid Calculi, 224

Valves, Posterior Urethral, 3-7, 105-108
Vesical Neck Contracture, 9-12
Vesicoureteral Reflux, 93-94
  Post TUR Bladder, 95-99, 109
  With Posterior Urethral Valves, 105-108

Wilms' Tumor, 178-183

Xanthogranulomatous Pyelonephritis, 116-119

Y-V Plasty, Bladder Neck, 11

POST-TEST

MULTIPLE CHOICE

1. A 15-year-old boy is seen with a history of sudden onset of pain in the right testicle of 12 hours duration. On examination, the right hemiscrotum is markedly enlarged, reddened and exquisitely tender. The scrotal contents cannot be adequately differentiated. The next treatment should be
   A. bed rest, scrotal elevation, and analgesics
   B. A, plus antibiotics
   C. immediate surgical exploration for possible torsion
   D. xylocaine block of cord for better examination

2. A 24-year-old male notices a firm lump in his right testicle which appears to be a tumor. Intravenous urogram, lymphangiogram, gonadotropin and alphafetoprotein are normal. Orchiectomy reveals pure seminoma. Further therapy should be
   A. none, since there is no evidence of metastases
   B. retroperitoneal lymph node dissection
   C. radiotherapy to the abdominal lymph nodes
   D. chemotherapy with VAB regimen

3. A 26-year-old male undergoes radical orchiectomy for a teratocarcinoma of the right testicle. After appropriate preoperative evaluation, a modified bilateral retroperitoneal lymph node dissection is performed. Thirty-three nodes are removed, and all are negative for tumor. Hormone assays are negative, and there is no evidence of metastatic disease. Therapy at this time should include
   A. treatment with DDP, vinblastine and bleomycin
   B. treatment with VAB regimen
   C. postoperative radiotherapy
   D. watchful waiting

4. An 18-year-old boy is seen because of a lump in his left testicle. Intravenous urogram is within normal limits. Lymphangiogram shows enlarged nodes with multiple filling defects in the left perihilar renal area. Alpha fetoprotein and

gonadotropins are elevated. Radical orchiectomy is performed, and an embryonal carcinoma is found. Further therapy should be
   A. chemotherapy with VAB regimen
   B. retroperitoneal lymph node dissection
   C. external radiotherapy
   D. percutaneous biopsy of lymph node

5. A retroperitoneal lymph node dissection is performed, and eight of forty-two nodes are positive - all in the area of the left renal vein. Chest x-ray is negative. There are no other signs of metastases. One would
   A. treat with post-op radiation
   B. treat with DDP, vinblastine and bleomycin
   C. perform mediastinal node dissection
   D. give radiation to abdomen and mediastinum and neck

6. Six months later, a chest x-ray revealed numerous nodules in both lung fields. The patient was given a course of DDP (cis-diaminodichloroplatinum), Velban and bleomycin, and all nodules disappeared completely, except one in the right upper lobe. One would
   A. give radiotherapy to lung
   B. add actinomycin D to regimen
   C. perform right upper lobe lobectomy
   D. abandon further treatment

7. Which of the following is not of germ cell origin?
   A. choriocarcinoma
   B. seminoma
   C. embryonal carcinoma
   D. orchioblastoma
   E. interstitial cell tumor

8. A 43-year-old male is seen because of a mass in his scrotum at the inferior border of the testicle. Intravenous urogram is normal. Hormone assays are normal. Exploration through an inguinal incision reveals a solid mass in the tail of the epididymis. Proper treatment would be
   A. radical orchiectomy
   B. biopsy of the lesion since the most likely diagnosis is benign. An epididymectomy should follow
   C. radical orchiectomy with retroperitoneal lymph node dissection
   D. epididymectomy only

9. The most reliable method of obtaining specimens of suspected prostatic carcinoma is
   A. needle biopsy
   B. transurethral prostatic resection
   C. open perineal biopsy
   D. transrectal needle biopsy
   E. enucleation prostatectomy

10. The initial site of nodal metastases in carcinoma of the prostate is
    A. external iliac nodes
    B. inguinal nodes
    C. obturator nodes
    D. presacral nodes
    E. common iliac nodes

11. Segmental resection of the bladder for carcinoma should be reserved for patients with
    A. high grade, low stage tumors
    B. low grade, low stage tumors
    C. no evidence of metastases
    D. tumors confined to the anterior wall and dome
    E. none of the above

12. The final common pathway of the chemical carcinogen in bladder tumors is
    A. 2-Naphthylamine
    B. Tryptophan
    C. ortho-amino-phenols
    D. beta-glucuronidase

13. Renal dysplasia can be found in which of the following?
    A. Ureterocele with duplication
    B. Ureteropelvic junction obstruction
    C. Multicystic kidney
    D. Congenital reflux
    E. All of the above

14. All of the following are true in relation to multicystic kidney, except
    A. it is almost always unilateral
    B. it is inherited by an autosomal recessive trait
    C. it is characterized by an irregular lobulated mass of cysts
    D. the ureter is usually atretic or absent

15. Fetal renal hamartoma, a benign tumor of the kidney, closely resembles
    A. neuroblastoma
    B. orchioblastoma
    C. Wilms' tumor
    D. renal cell carcinoma
    E. liposarcoma

16. The chemotherapeutic drug of choice in Wilms' tumor of the kidney is
    A. vincristine
    B. 5-Fluorouracil
    C. actinomycin D
    D. bleomycin
    E. A & C

17. Angiomyolipoma of the kidney is frequently associated with
    A. tuberculosis
    B. multiple endocrine tumors
    C. tuberous sclerosis
    D. myelofibrosis

18. The treatment of choice for malignant neoplasm of the distal end of the ureter is
    A. excision of the tumor with at least 2cm of normal ureter proximally and distally, and end-to-end ureteroureterostomy
    B. nephroureterectomy
    C. excision of distal ureter and reimplantation into bladder
    D. nephroureterectomy with a cuff of bladder

19. Which of the following is the most helpful in the preoperative diagnosis of transitional cell carcinoma of the renal pelvis?
    A. Urine cytology from the affected kidney
    B. Renal angiogram
    C. Infusion intravenous urogram
    D. Nephrotomography
    E. CAT scan

20. All of the following should be removed at the time of radical nephrectomy, except
    A. Gerota's fat and fascia
    B. the ipsilateral adrenal gland
    C. the lymph nodes, from the crus of the diaphragm, to the bifurcation of the aorta
    D. the entire ureter

21. Abnormal liver chemistries (elevated SGOT, SGPT, bilirubin and alkaline phosphatase), when found preoperatively in renal cell carcinoma, indicate
    A. a poor prognosis
    B. a liver biopsy should be done
    C. concomitant hepatic disease is present
    D. B & C
    E. nothing of prognostic value

22. A 36-year-old male is seen in the emergency room after being in an automobile accident. He has gross total hematuria. An intravenous urogram shows some delay in excretion on the left side, but a normal collecting system with a small amount of extravasation of contrast material. A left renal angiogram is normal. Proper therapy would include
    A. exploring left kidney and draining retroperitoneum
    B. passing a left ureteral catheter
    C. watchful waiting
    D. performing a left nephrectomy

23. You are called to the operating room by one of your surgical colleagues, who tells you that he had just accidentally ligated the right ureter in its distal third. After removal of the ligature, it is noted to be pale, and peristalsis is absent. What would the procedure of choice be?
    A. Reimplantation into bladder
    B. Transureteroureterostomy
    C. Nephroureterectomy
    D. Excision of ligated ureter and reanastomosis
    E. No further treatment is necessary at this time

24. A 40-year-old female is seen because of gross total painless hematuria. She denies any other urinary symptoms or problems. Plain film of the abdomen shows a Staghorn calculus of the left kidney. Intravenous urogram shows a normal right kidney, a good nephrogram on the left with good excretion. One would perform
    A. left nephrectomy
    B. left nephrolithotomy
    C. watchful waiting
    D. antibiotic prophylaxis
    E. hydration therapy

25. A 55-year-old female is seen for gross hematuria. Intravenous urogram shows a solitary left kidney with a mass at the lower pole. Angiogram reveals a tumor of the lower

pole. BUN and creatinine are normal. There is no evidence of metastases. Proper therapy would be
   A. radical nephrectomy followed by chronic dialysis
   B. radical nephrectomy and transplantation when a donor becomes available
   C. lower pole partial nephrectomy
   D. chemotherapy
   E. external radiotherapy

26. A 58-year-old male undergoes transurethral resection of the prostate. Two chips show adenocarcinoma. Acid phosphatase is normal, and there is no evidence of metastatic disease. Proper therapy would be
   A. radical prostatectomy by perineal route
   B. retropubic radical prostatectomy and lymph node dissection
   C. external radiotherapy
   D. lymph node dissection and I^{125} implants
   E. watchful waiting

27. Alpha-adrenergic stimulation of the bladder
   A. decreases outlet resistance
   B. increases intraurethral pressure
   C. is produced by phenoxybenzamine
   D. produces relaxation of the detrusor
   E. causes contraction of smooth muscle at the bladder neck

28. All of the following are characteristic of bladder dysfunction, secondary to a lesion of the sacral cord, except
   A. low intravesical pressure
   B. large capacity bladder
   C. involuntary detrusor contraction
   D. decreased sphincter tone
   E. bladder trabeculations

29. In the acutely injured spinal cord patient, the initial phase of urologic management is best handled by
   A. Foley catheter drainage with intermittent irrigation
   B. Foley catheter drainage with continuous bladder irrigation
   C. intermittent catheterization
   D. suprapubic cystostomy
   E. allowing patient to void spontaneously

30. Which of the following are frequently helpful in attaining bladder emptying in suprasacral cord lesions?
    A. Bethanechol
    B. Ephedrine
    C. Sphincterotomy
    D. Pro-Banthine
    E. A & C

31. All of the neurologic findings below are associated with suprasacral cord lesions, except
    A. frequent upper urinary tract deterioration
    B. uninhibited bladder contractions
    C. spasticity of external sphincter
    D. decreased bladder capacity
    E. absence of bulbocavernosus reflex

32. All of the neurologic conditions below are associated with interruption of Loop I pathways to the bladder, except
    A. stroke
    B. brain tumor
    C. Parkinson's disease
    D. spinal cord tumor
    E. dementia

33. The optimum incision for a pheochromocytoma would be
    A. thoraco-abdominal
    B. classical flank
    C. through the twelfth rib
    D. anterior transperitoneal midline

34. The preferred method of radiographic demonstration of an adrenal tumor is
    A. renal artery angiography
    B. nephrotomography
    C. adrenal venography
    D. presacral CO_2 insufflation
    E. sonography

35. If the renal artery is to be clamped without renal cooling, ischemia time should not exceed
    A. 10 minutes
    B. 20 minutes
    C. 30 minutes
    D. 60 minutes
    E. 120 minutes

36. The mechanism of action of allopurinol primarily
    A. increases urinary pH
    B. decreases uric acid excretion
    C. decreases uric acid production
    D. increases solubility of uric acid

37. The most common type of renal calculus in the United States is
    A. uric acid
    B. magnesium ammonium phosphate
    C. calcium carbonate
    D. calcium oxalate
    E. phosphate stone

MATCH EACH OF THE NUMBERED ITEMS WITH THE APPROPRIATE LETTERED ITEMS

38. ___ Penis   A. Mesonephric duct
39. ___ Uterus   B. Genital tubercle
40. ___ Ureter   C. Mullerian duct
41. ___ Appendix testis   D. Metanephric bud
42. ___ Paraoophoron   E. Urogenital sinus
43. ___ Prostate   F. Wolffian duct

44. A 45-year-old female is 7 days postvaginal hysterectomy, and found to be leaking urine per vagina from a vesicovaginal fistula. Treatment of choice would be
    A. immediate closure of fistula by vaginal route
    B. immediate fulguration of the fistula
    C. Foley catheter drainage for 3 months
    D. observation for 3 months, and repair of fistula at that time if healing does not occur
    E. suprapubic cystostomy

45. A 30-year-old female is seen because of right renal colic and hematuria. Plain film of the abdomen reveals a 4mm x 4mm calculus at L4. Intravenous urogram shows Grade II hydro-ureteronephrosis down to this point. She is asymptomatic. One would
    A. pass a ureteral catheter
    B. continue observation
    C. perform ureterolithotomy
    D. perform cystoscopy and ureteral stone basket extraction

46. A 30-year-old male undergoes right ureterolithotomy of a low ureteral calculus. Fifteen days later, there is still copious urinary leakage from the drain site. Intravenous urogram shows a mild hydroureteronephrosis down to the

operative site, with extravasation at that point. The lower ureter is never seen. What would one do?
A. Pass a ureteral catheter
B. Perform ureteral reimplantation into the bladder, if feasible
C. Perform transureteroureterostomy
D. Merely repair the open ureter
E. Watchful waiting is called for at this point

47. Clinical findings associated with renal cell carcinoma can include
A. fever
B. hypercalcemia
C. polycythemia
D. amyloidosis
E. all of the above

48. Nephrectomy for renal tuberculosis is indicated
A. in severe cases with a normal contralateral kidney
B. in a nonfunctioning kidney
C. to cure the patient completely
D. in all of the above
E. rarely, if ever

49. The earliest pyelographic evidence of tuberculosis is
A. ureteral stricture with obstruction
B. calcification in the renal parenchyma
C. papillary destruction with irregularity of the minor calyx
D. infundibular scarring

50. With minimal involvement of the kidney, and the presence of a positive urine culture for M. tuberculosis, the preferred method of management would be
A. streptomycin, INH, and PAS
B. two drugs are as good as three
C. ethambutol, INH, and cycloserine
D. INH for 2 years

51. Calculi following papillary necrosis are characterized by which of the following?
A. "Jackstone" type
B. "Waxy" appearance
C. Radiolucent center and radiopaque periphery
D. Attachment to papilla
E. Complete radiolucency

52. Which of the following are not etiologic factors in papillary necrosis?
    A. Diabetes
    B. Chronic pyelonephritis
    C. Sickle cell trait
    D. Phenacetin ingestion
    E. None of the above

MATCH EACH OF THE NUMBERED ITEMS WITH THE APPROPRIATE LETTERED ITEMS

53. ___ Inulin   A. Glomerular function
54. ___ Mannitol   B. Tubular function
55. ___ PAH   C. Renal blood flow
56. ___ I^{131}-orthoiodohippurate

57. A diverticulum is differentiated from bladder on cystogram by which of the following?
    A. Diverticulum is always smaller
    B. Diverticulum is always larger
    C. Diverticulum is smooth
    D. Diverticulum is "scalloped"
    E. None of the above

58. Carcinoma of the prostate is most commonly found in the
    A. lateral lobes
    B. middle lobe
    C. subcervical lobe
    D. anterior lobe
    E. posterior lobe

59. The ectopic ureterocele is usually found in
    A. the upper segment of a duplex kidney
    B. the lower segment of a duplex kidney
    C. an ectopic kidney
    D. a solitary kidney

60. Y-V plasty of ureteropelvic junction obstruction should be reserved exclusively for
    A. vessel at ureteropelvic junction
    B. high insertion of ureter
    C. mucosal valve causing obstruction
    D. extrinsic scar formation
    E. adynamic pelvis

61. Hydronephrosis can be differentiated from neoplasm of the kidney in children by
    A. transillumination
    B. firmness of the mass
    C. irregularity of the mass
    D. extension of the mass across the midline
    E. all of the above

62. The majority of urethral strictures is best treated by
    A. Johansen urethroplasty
    B. Devine procedure
    C. urethral dilatations
    D. Turner-Warwick urethroplasty
    E. Blandy urethroplasty

63. Urinary extravasation in blunt renal trauma requires which of the following?
    A. Immediate surgery and drainage
    B. Immediate repair of renal injury
    C. Is not in and of itself an indication for surgery
    D. Nephrectomy
    E. Passage of a ureteral catheter

64. Proper therapy for a severed ureter discovered during the course of a hysterectomy would be
    A. ligation of ureter
    B. ureteroureterostomy
    C. transureteroureterostomy
    D. ureteroneocystostomy
    E. nephrectomy

65. A 35-year-old female undergoes abdominal hysterectomy, and on the tenth postoperative day, develops fever of 103° and right flank pain. An intravenous urogram shows Grade IV hydroureteronephrosis on the right. Proper therapy would be
    A. immediate right nephrostomy
    B. immediate right nephrectomy
    C. cystoscopy and ureteral catheterization
    D. exploration and ureteroureterostomy
    E. none of the above

66. Ureterovaginal fistula is best diagnosed by
    A. intravenous indigo carmine
    B. intravesical indigo carmine
    C. intravenous urogram
    D. B plus A
    E. all of the above

67. In a gunshot would of the abdomen involving both bladder and rectosigmoid, proper therapy should include
    A. colostomy
    B. suprapubic cystostomy
    C. interposition of omentum between bladder and bowel
    D. drainage of perivesical space
    E. all of the above

68. A urethral injury which penetrates Buck's fascia could show
    A. extravasation into the scrotum
    B. extravasation into the perineum
    C. edema of the penis
    D. extravasation onto the abdominal wall
    E. all of the above

69. The cardinal sign of anterior urethral injury is
    A. hematoma of penis
    B. tenderness in the perineum
    C. blood from the urethral meatus
    D. inability to void
    E. dysuria after "straddle injury"

70. Perinephric abscess is generally found
    A. beneath the renal capsule, and outside the renal parenchyma
    B. between renal capsule and Gerota's fascia
    C. outside Gerota's fascia
    D. from the collecting system into the renal parenchyma

MATCH EACH OF THE NUMBERED ITEMS WITH THE APPROPRIATE LETTERED ITEMS

71. ___ Oxybutynin   A. Detrusor stimulation
72. ___ Phenoxybenzamine   B. Bladder neck stimulation
73. ___ Bethanechol   C. Skeletal muscle relaxant
74. ___ Ephedrine   D. Detrusor relaxation
75. ___ Dantrolene   E. Bladder neck relaxation

76. A 63-year-old male has a transurethral resection of papillary bladder tumor. Pathology report is Grade II transitional carcinoma with no muscle invasion. There is no evidence of metastasis. Further treatment would be
    A. cystectomy and ileal loop diversion
    B. intracavitary radiotherapy
    C. external radiotherapy
    D. cystoscopy every 3 months for 2 years
    E. intravesical thio-tepa

77. A 3-year-old girl is seen because of recurrent urinary tract infection with a temperature of 103°. She responds rapidly to a course of ampicillin. Intravenous urogram is normal. Cystogram shows reflux into the entire right kidney. Cystoscopy is normal. Proper therapy would be
    A. long-term antibiotic therapy
    B. right ureteral reimplantation
    C. treatment for 10 days with ampicillin and observation
    D. bilateral ureteral reimplantation

78. A 61-year-old male undergoes a transurethral resection of the prostate. Pathologic report shows infiltrating adenocarcinoma in many of the chips. He is in good condition. Proper therapy would be
    A. observation only
    B. radical prostatectomy
    C. megavoltage radiotherapy
    D. bilateral orchiectomy
    E. B or C

79. A 60-year-old male undergoes transurethral resection of multiple bladder tumors. Pathology report is Grade IV transitional cell carcinoma with muscle invasion. There is no evidence of metastatic disease. Therapy would be
    A. recystoscopy every 3 months for 2 years
    B. radical cystectomy
    C. external radiotherapy
    D. preoperative radiotherapy and radical cystectomy
    E. intracavitary radiation

80. A 50-year-old male is brought to the emergency room after being struck by an automobile. There is gross bleeding from his urethra. He cannot void. An intravenous urogram shows multiple pelvic fractures, normal kidneys. The bladder is high in the pelvis, and compressed to a "tear drop" shape. Proper initial therapy would be
    A. passing a urethral catheter
    B. performing a urethrogram
    C. performing a suprapubic cystostomy
    D. re-establishing urethral continuity by immediate surgery

ANSWER QUESTIONS 81-90 USING THE FOLLOWING KEY

   A. If both statement and reason are true and related cause and effect
   B. If both statement and reason are true but not related cause and effect
   C. If the statement is true, but the reason false
   D. If the statement is false, but the reason true
   E. If both statement and reason are false

81. A perinephric abscess may present just above the iliac crest posterolaterally BECAUSE the space between Gerota's fascia and the kidney extends inferiorly to this area.

82. The degree of hematuria is an important sign in renal injury BECAUSE the degree of hematuria correlates directly with the degree of injury.

83. The conservative management of most renal injuries has become the treatment of choice BECAUSE antibiotic therapy has decreased the incidence of infection.

84. It is important to rule out vesicoureteral reflux prior to surgery for ureteropelvic junction obstruction BECAUSE reflux can sometimes be an etiologic factor in obstruction.

85. Cytologic examination of the urine is helpful in the follow-up of patients with low grade bladder tumors BECAUSE one can detect early recurrences of bladder tumors by urine cytology.

86. All scrotal masses should be explored surgically BECAUSE the majority of scrotal masses are malignant.

87. Injuries to the bladder by a direct blow generally result in intraperitoneal tears BECAUSE the weakest point of the full bladder is at the dome beneath the peritoneal reflection.

88. Following prostatectomy for benign disease, the development of carcinoma is rare BECAUSE most of the tumorogenic prostate is removed with enucleation prostatectomy.

89. Filling of the bladder is said to be related to sympathetic innervation, and emptying to parasympathetic innervation

BECAUSE stimulation of sympathetic pathways causes relaxation of the body of the bladder and constriction of fibers at the bladder neck.

90. Xanthogranulomatous pyelonephritis can rarely be confused with renal cell carcinoma BECAUSE xanthogranulomatous pyelonephritis has giant histiocytes on histologic sections.

ANSWER TRUE OR FALSE FOR QUESTIONS 91-96

91. Staging of bladder tumors can be accurately accomplished by transurethral resection.

92. Calcification around the periphery of a renal mass is indicative of renal cyst in 95% of cases.

93. Central, stippled calcification within a renal mass indicates neoplasm in many cases.

94. Most staghorn calculi are asymptomatic.

95. Because most staghorn calculi are asymptomatic, it is better to leave them alone as long as they are non-obstructive.

96. The most common organism associated with infected staghorn calculi is E. coli.

MATCH EACH OF THE NUMBERED ITEMS WITH THE APPROPRIATE LETTERED ITEMS

97. ___ Uric acid
98. ___ Cystine
99. ___ Magnesium ammonium phosphate
100. ___ Calcium oxalate

A. Jackstones
B. Proteus species
C. Radiolucent
D. Inherited disorder

101. All of the following are associated with hypercalcemia, except
    A. sarcoidosis
    B. multiple myeloma
    C. hyperparathyroidism
    D. renal cell carcinoma
    E. peptic ulcer

102. A 6-month-old male child is seen because of recurrent urinary tract infections. An intravenous urogram shows massively dilated upper urinary tracts. Voiding cystourethrogram reveals bilateral vesicoureteral reflux and posterior urethral valves. BUN and creatinine are normal, and, at present, the child is uninfected. Initial therapy should be
    A. bilateral cutaneous ureterostomies
    B. suprapubic cystostomy
    C. resection of valves transurethrally
    D. Foley catheter drainage until the upper tracts improve
    E. bilateral nephrostomy

ANSWER KEY

The author has made every effort to thoroughly verify the answers to the questions which appear on the preceding pages. However, as in any text, some inaccuracies and ambiguities may occur; therefore, if in doubt, please consult standard references.

THE PUBLISHER

1.	C	27.	E	53.	A	79.	D
2.	C	28.	C	54.	A	80.	C
3.	D	29.	C	55.	B	81.	A
4.	B	30.	C	56.	C	82.	E
5.	D	31.	E	57.	C	83.	B
6.	C	32.	D	58.	E	84.	A
7.	E	33.	D	59.	A	85.	D
8.	B	34.	C	60.	B	86.	E
9.	C	35.	C	61.	A	87.	A
10.	C	36.	C	62.	C	88.	E
11.	D	37.	D	63.	C	89.	A
12.	C	38.	B	64.	D	90.	D
13.	E	39.	C	65.	C	91.	F
14.	B	40.	D	66.	D	92.	F
15.	C	41.	C	67.	E	93.	T
16.	E	42.	F	68.	E	94.	F
17.	C	43.	E	69.	C	95.	F
18.	D	44.	D	70.	B	96.	F
19.	C	45.	B	71.	D	97.	C
20.	D	46.	A	72.	E	98.	D
21.	E	47.	E	73.	A	99.	B
22.	C	48.	E	74.	B	100.	A
23.	A	49.	C	75.	C	101.	E
24.	B	50.	C	76.	D	102.	C
25.	C	51.	C	77.	A		
26.	E	52.	E	78.	E		